Pregnancy
How to look good and feel great

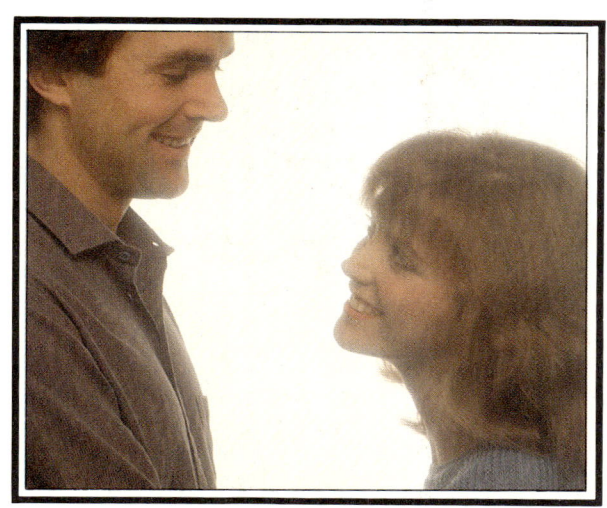

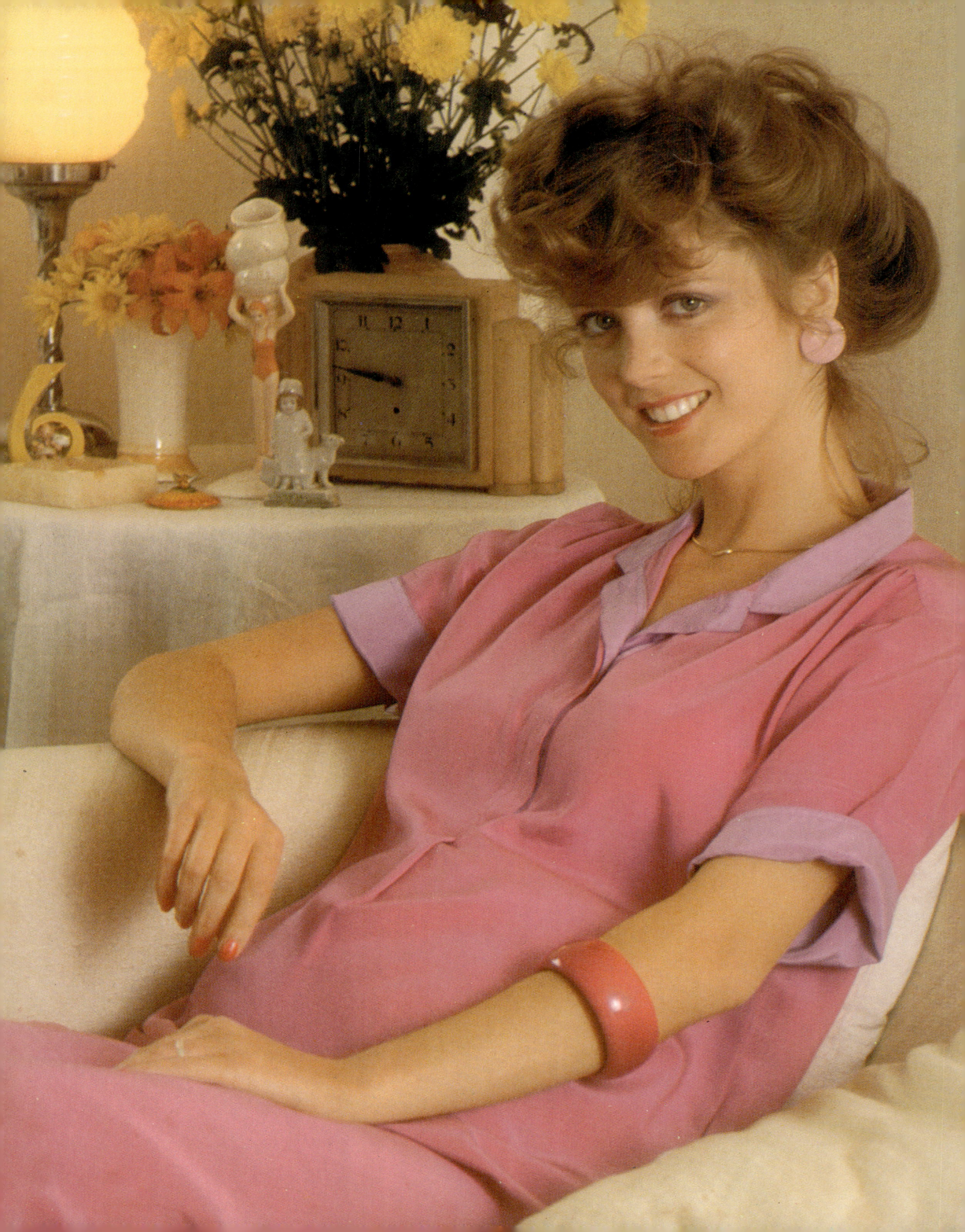

Pregnancy

How to look good and feel great

Bonnie Estridge and Mary Lou

TREASURE PRESS

For Giles and Hannah

First published in Great Britain in 1982 by Artus Publishing Company Ltd

This edition published in 1985 by Treasure Press 59 Grosvenor Street London W1

© **1982 Bonnie Estridge and Mary Lou**

ISBN 1 85051 041 5

Printed in Hong Kong

Design and art direction by Kieran Stevens Photography by Chris Holland, Tom Leighton and Peter Meyers

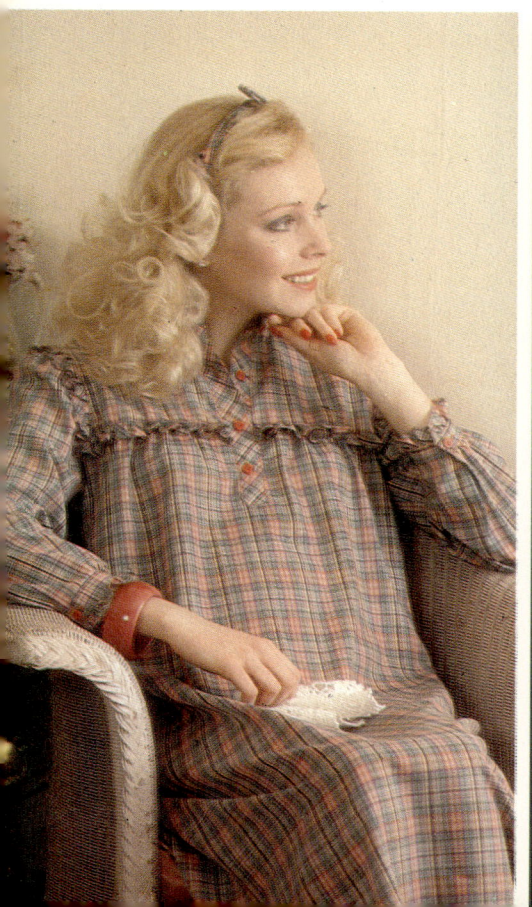
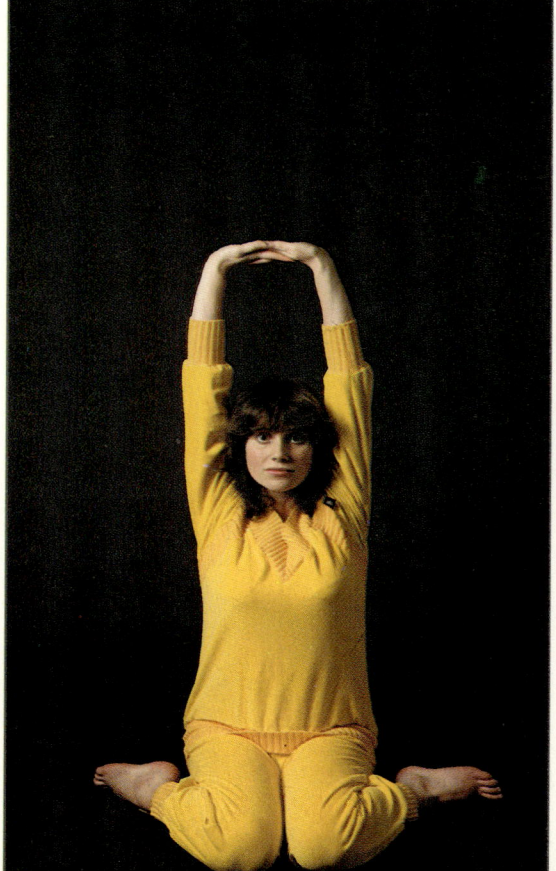
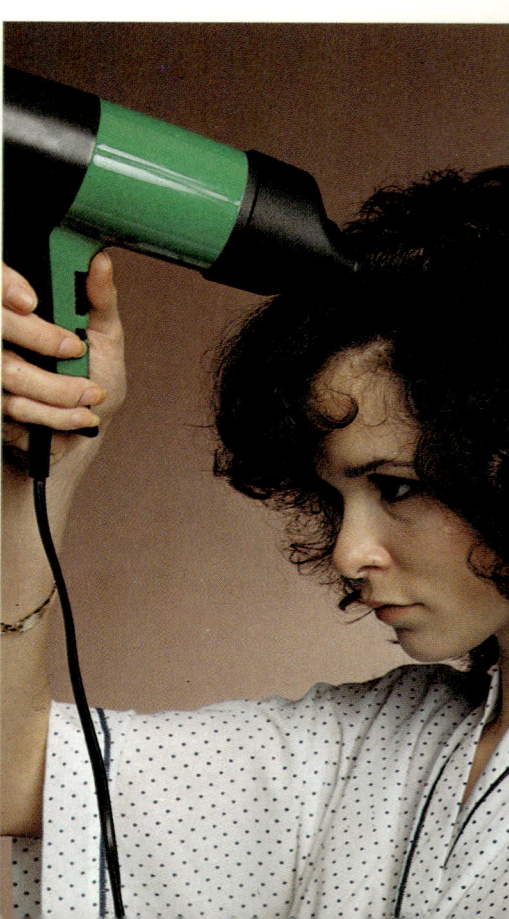

Contents

Introduction	7
The Beginning of Your Pregnancy	8
You and Your Emotions	14
Body Care	24
Exercise	30
Diet and Weight	38
Skin and Make-up	48
Hair	54
Fashion	60
Family and Household	72
When the Big Day Arrives	76
Index	80

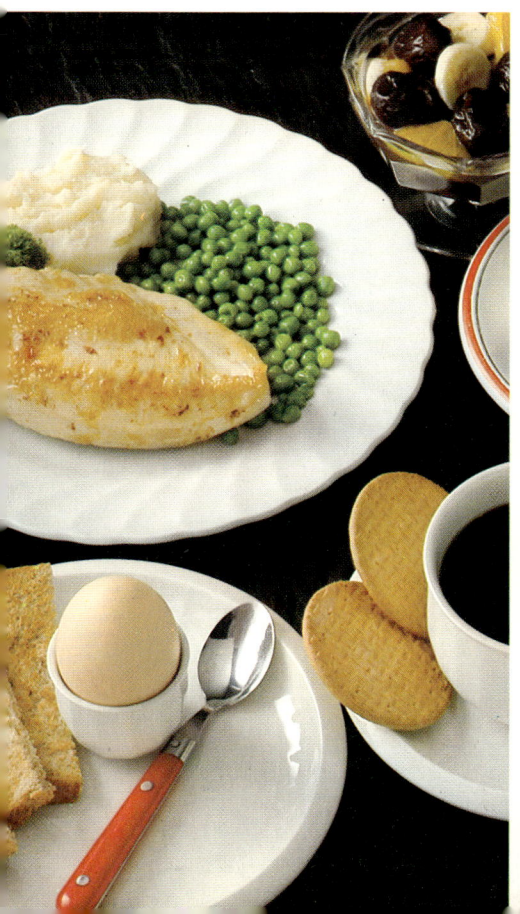

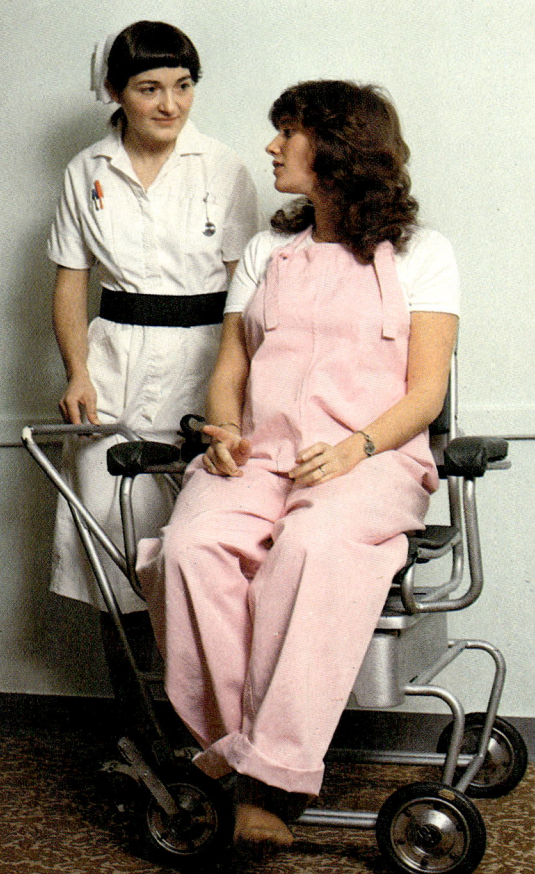

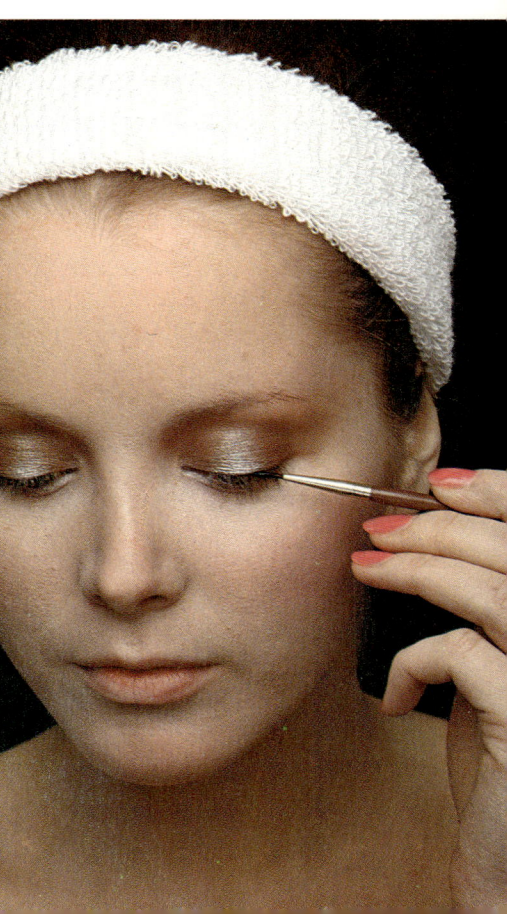

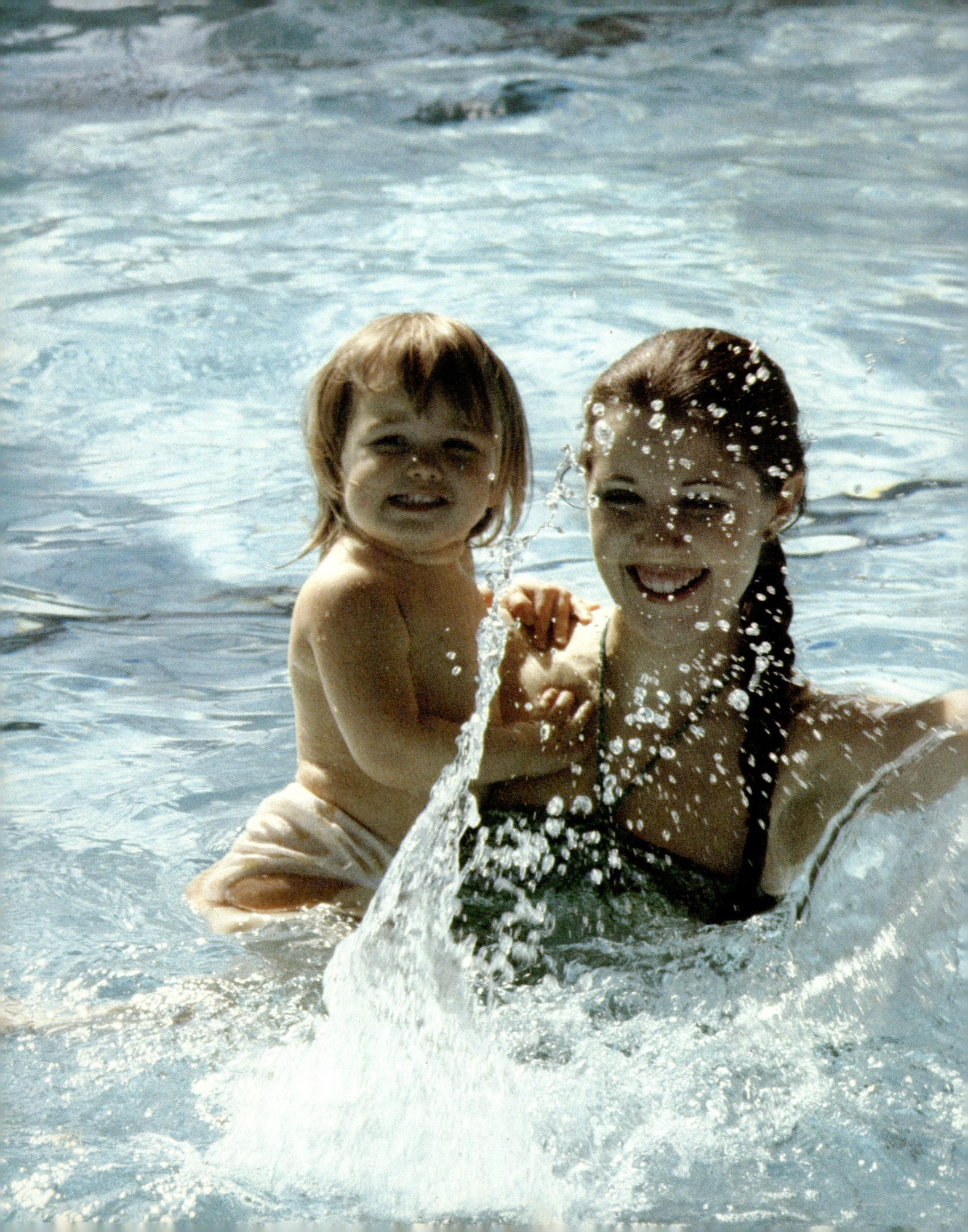

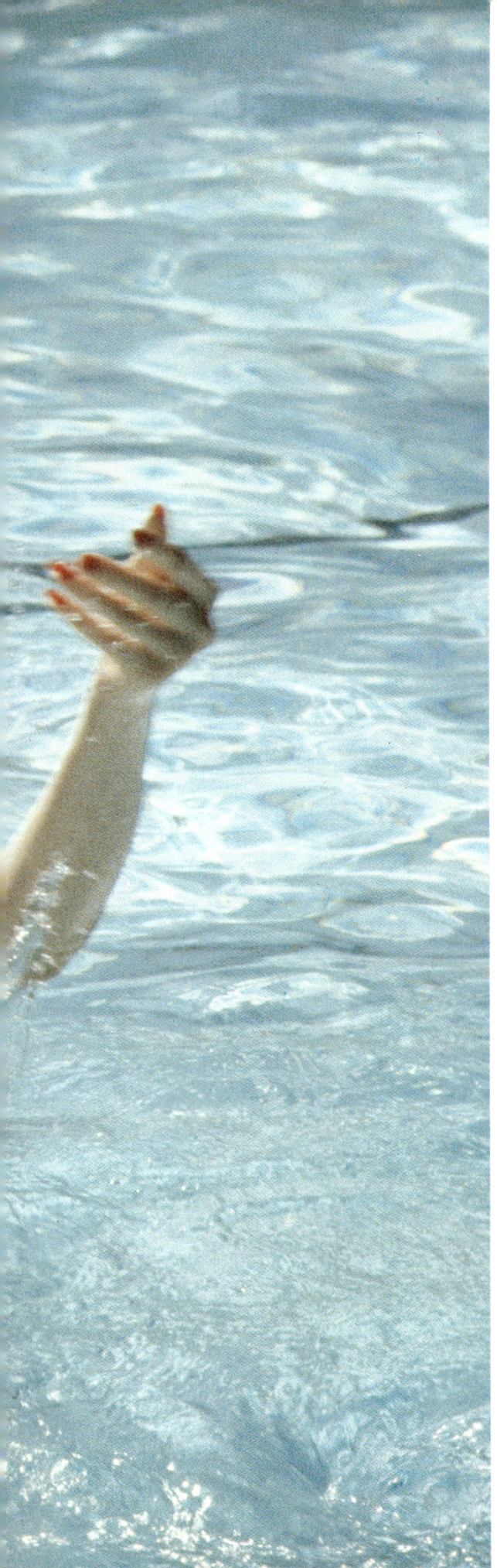

Introduction

Most books on pregnancy have a strong medical bias, and though they may tackle every physical detail from the development of the baby to what to do if your nose bleeds, they tend to say little or nothing about the way a pregnant woman feels about herself – the emotional changes, fears, depressions and elations that commonly or uncommonly occur. Generally the assumption seems to be that everyone has a carbon copy pregnancy. This is far from true. Each individual and each pregnancy is unique, and people react quite differently to the experience. Everyone expects you to feel happy and wonderful, but there are times when you just feel depressed about the way you look and wonder how you'll ever be able to get through the weeks of waiting.

We were both pregnant when we wrote this book, and we quickly discovered that medical guides don't offer much practical advice on beauty, fashion or body care for the pregnant woman – how she can cope with her appearance and changing shape and make the most of her natural, very feminine state without looking dowdy. Do not despair as your body changes, instead try a new hairstyle to suit your new shape, and adapt your normal make-up routine to make the most of that bloom. Looking good is a great psychological boost. There's no need to dress like a walking tent, there are fashions available that flatter but are comfortable too.

Body care is very important during pregnancy. Many women ignore exercise until after the birth, when it may be too late. If you follow our simple but effective exercise programme, you should feel fitter and more relaxed as well as keeping your muscles in tone for the delivery and afterwards, when you want to get your figure back quickly.

The chances are you will have a trouble-free pregnancy – the majority of women do. Our aim is to minimize the problems should they arise and to help you feel good about yourself, so that you can make the most of a very personal experience.

The Beginning of your Pregnancy

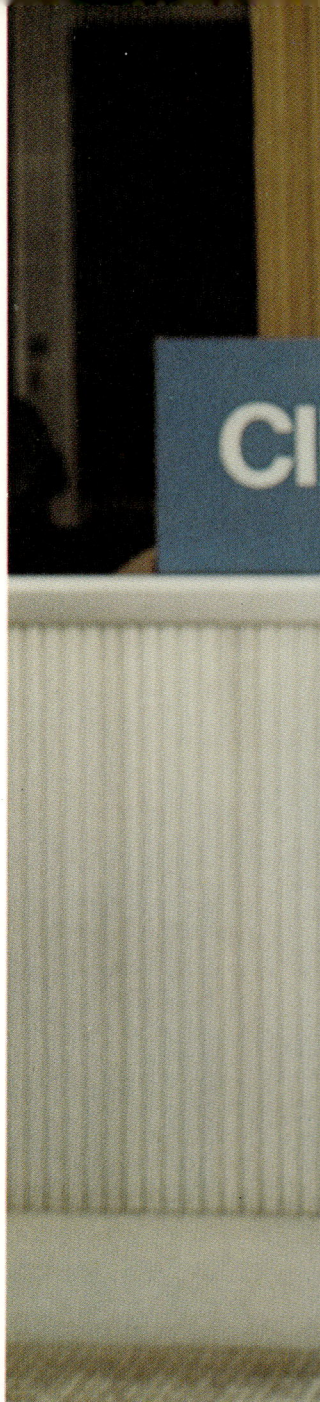

Although we always think of a pregnancy as lasting nine calendar months, the length of time for an average pregnancy is actually ten lunar months. The date of delivery is calculated as forty weeks from the first day of your last period, which means around 280 days of waiting. At the beginning of your pregnancy the weeks stretching ahead will feel like an eternity. But however far away the birth might seem you should make preparations for it right from the start. It is important to take the time and trouble to understand what is happening to your body – you will feel far more confident if you do and probably enjoy your pregnancy more.

Confirming your pregnancy

Missing one period is not sufficient evidence to be certain that you are pregnant. You may have other early signs – sore breasts, feeling extra tired, needing to pass urine more frequently, nausea. To be sure, you should have a simple urine test six weeks from the first day of your last period. Take an early morning urine sample (i.e. one taken before you have eaten or drunk anything) to your doctor or family planning clinic, or to a chemist who performs these tests. Most chemists are able to give you an answer in ten minutes, the doctor or clinic may take a while longer. If you can't wait to find out there are home-testing kits on the market which, if you use them carefully and according to the instructions, will give you a reliable result. But do have this confirmed by a clinical test afterwards just to be certain. A positive result is accurate in over ninety-nine per cent of cases, but a negative result does not necessarily mean that you are not pregnant. The pregnancy test detects the presence or absence of the hormone chorionic gonadotrophin in the urine (the first hormone produced by the pregnancy and initially responsible for maintaining it). If the test has been performed too early there may not be a sufficiently high level of this hormone to give a positive result. Therefore, if you do have a negative result but feel sure that you are pregnant, wait for a week and then have another test.

Pregnancy can also be detected by a vaginal examination to feel if the uterus is enlarged, although this method isn't a hundred per cent reliable. Alternatively, you can have an ultrasound scan (using high frequency sound waves), which is harmless and very accurate, but more generally used to monitor the baby's progress rather than to diagnose pregnancy.

Antenatal care

As soon as you have a positive result, go and see your doctor or obstetrician and discuss with him the arrangements that you want made for care during your pregnancy and delivery. If this is your first baby you will probably prefer to have a hospital confinement, whether in a private or National Health Service hospital, rather than opt for a home birth – indeed your doctor will almost certainly recommend this. He will tell you which hospital to attend for antenatal care. You may be referred to a General Practitioner Maternity Unit if you have one in your area; these are usually attached to a large hospital so that every facility is available. Alternatively he may look after you himself.

Book into the hospital early and start antenatal check-ups from about the eighth week to ensure that everything goes smoothly from an early stage. Antenatal check-ups are usually monthly until twenty-eight weeks, then fortnightly until the last month when you will be asked to attend the clinic or doctor's surgery every week. On your first antenatal visit your doctor or midwife will ask you for details of your family and medical history, of any previous pregnancies, and will also need information about the suitability of your accommodation if you are planning to have your baby at home. After the interview you will have a general medical examination plus a vaginal examination and a blood test.

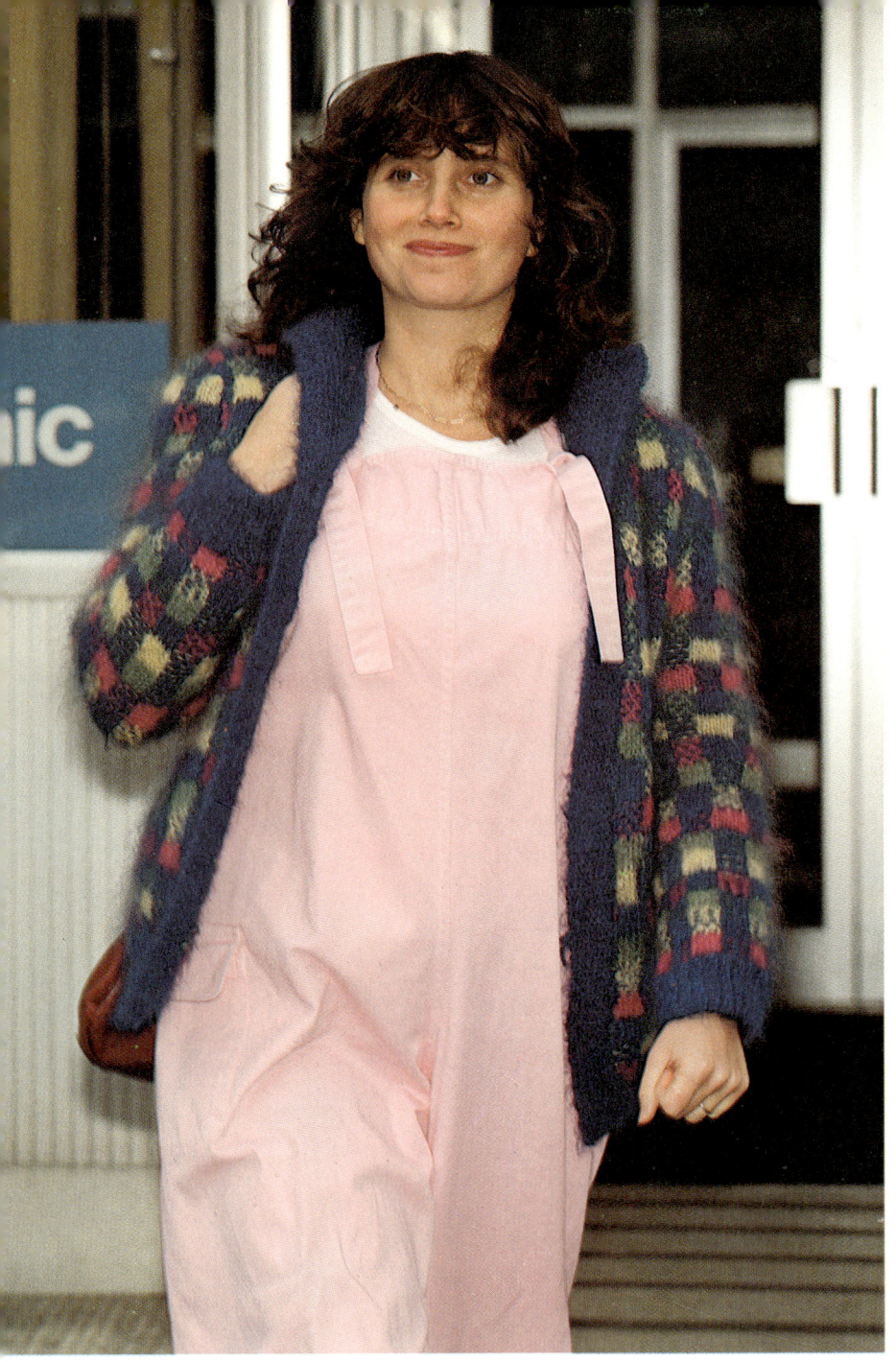

Hospital clinics

Some women find hospital maternity units bustling, unfriendly places where they are made to feel like an anonymous number. This is a pity as each visit to the antenatal clinic is an exciting step nearer to the baby being born. You should bear in mind though that hospital staff tend to be busy and overworked and if everything is straightforward they may refrain from giving you information unless you ask. The majority of doctors and their staff are only too pleased to answer your questions and allay your fears, but they can't be expected to mind read. So, if you do have questions it's a good idea to make a list of them and keep it handy so that you make the best use of limited time.

It will also make things easier for you and the hospital staff if you dress sensibly when you go to the clinic. This may sound trivial, but doctors have been known to complain of pregnant ladies struggling to get their boots off for the weighing machine or wearing tight sleeves that won't roll up the arm far enough for a blood pressure check. In general, a sympathetic understanding of the problems that harassed staff in overcrowded clinics have to face will help you to enjoy your hospital visits more and to put up cheerfully with the inevitable delays.

Booking up classes

Many hospitals with maternity units run antenatal mothercraft classes, which teach relaxation techniques and give general guidance on pregnancy and labour. They will also cover the essential things you will need to know when the baby is born, such as breast and bottle feeding, and nappy changing. Most classes include a film or slideshow of a home or hospital delivery to which prospective fathers are invited. The National Childbirth Trust, a private foundation with branches all over the country, holds classes on special breathing techniques that can be performed during labour and which help you to experience a relaxed birth with little or no help from drugs. Whichever type of course you choose, make sure that you enrol well in advance. Classes usually start six or eight weeks before your estimated delivery date and although this will seem a long way off when you are only twelve weeks pregnant, don't put it off because they invariably get booked up very quickly.

To help ensure a problem-free pregnancy, attend regular antenatal check-ups from an early stage, and make arrangements for the delivery as soon as your pregnancy has been confirmed.

A dietitian should be available to advise you on your diet during pregnancy and your midwife or doctor will tell you about breast care. If you have any social problems – if you are a single parent or have an accommodation problem, for example – you will be given the opportunity to see a medical social worker. On subsequent visits your weight, blood pressure, urine content and the general development of the baby will be checked and recorded until your confinement.

If you are going to have your baby at home, your G.P. and local domiciliary midwife (with whom your doctor will put you in touch immediately) will be jointly responsible for your antenatal care.

Immunization, drugs and pain-killers

On your first visit to the antenatal clinic or your doctor's surgery, a sample of blood will be taken to see if you are immune to German measles, which is one of the few organisms that can directly affect the foetus. If it is found that you don't have the necessary antibodies, you will *not* be given a vaccination against the infection. This is because the vaccine itself can damage the baby in the same way as the virus during the first twelve to fourteen weeks of pregnancy. However you will be advised to be immunized as soon after you have had the baby as possible. Meanwhile, you should keep well clear of anyone who has been in contact with the illness.

While you are pregnant, it is particularly important to follow your doctor's advice on is the use of drugs. If you already have a medical condition that requires the regular use of drugs your doctor will know whether it is safe to continue with these or whether they should be changed. For simple aches and pains paracetamol, aspirin and codeine are generally regarded as safe when taken in the prescribed dose, but avoid proprietary brands incorporating other chemicals or compounds, and always drink lots of fluid when taking the tablets. Alkalis taken for indigestion and heartburn are also harmless if taken in the prescribed dose. Some antibiotics however have an adverse effect on the growing baby and you should never take any medicines that have not been prescribed for you. As a general rule, avoid all drugs during pregnancy and, as a safety measure, check with your doctor before taking anything.

Antenatal classes cover the various kinds of drugs and aids that are available for labour, including psychoprophylaxis – the National Childbirth Trust's method of mental preparation and breathing; gas and air – a short-term analgesic you control yourself; pethidine – a long-lasting and more controversial pain-killer, which tends to make the baby sleepy too; and the increasingly popular epidural block – a local anaesthetic injected into the spinal canal, which gives very good pain relief while you still remain conscious to experience the birth. If your hospital performs the epidural they may ask you at the booking-in clinic whether you are going to want it, but there is really no need to make your mind up at this early stage.

You and your baby– step by step

The first three months
Many women suspect that they are pregnant some days before their period is due. Tingling, heaviness and soreness of the breasts are common symptoms. Queasiness, if not actual vomiting, and a general bloated feeling are also possible signs. But even if you do not become aware of your pregnancy at this stage the first weeks are the most important for the baby, which is developing rapidly from a fertilized egg into a foetus.

The egg is visible to the naked eye by the beginning of the second month. The spine, brain, heart and rudimentary organs are forming, the head growing faster than the body. By the end of this month limb buds are distinguishable, and the foetus is about 13 mm ($\frac{1}{2}$ in.) long.

By the start of the third month the foetus is recognizably human and is beginning to uncurl from its tight ball-like position, by the end of the month he measures around 7.5 cm (3 in.). If he has reached thirteen weeks without mishap, his chance of surviving to a live birth is very great.

At this stage you may still be feeling slightly sick or vomiting, or feeling tired, or needing to pass urine more than usual as the enlarging uterus starts to press on your bladder. By the end of the third month you will probably begin to put on some weight and find that your clothes are feeling tight, even though you can still wear them.

The fourth month
If you felt tired and nauseous for the first three months of pregnancy you should now feel better and brighter, and you will also be beginning to show. Between the thirteenth and eighteenth week your womb enlarges considerably and whereas the 'bump' was only just noticeable above your pubic bone at the beginning of the fourth month, by the end of this month it will have reached almost halfway to your navel.

During this month the foetus doubles its length from 7.5 cm (3 in.) to about 16 cm (6–7 in.) and is already kicking, although you are unlikely to feel these small, weak movements, especially if this is your first child. The baby's head will still be large in relation to the rest of its body but he is beginning to look more like a person – even the fingernails and toenails are starting to grow. By the end of this period the baby's sex will be determinable.

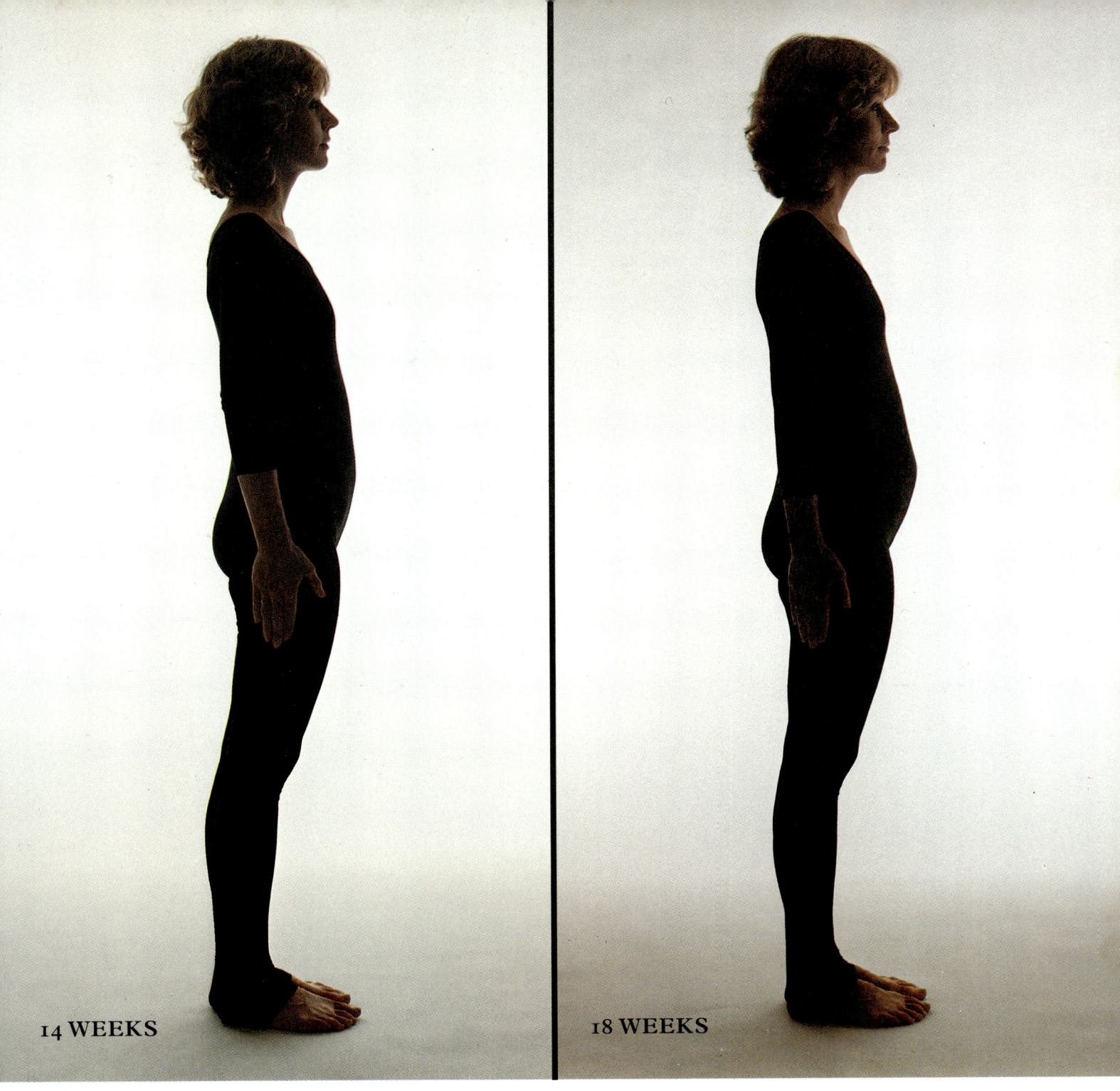

14 WEEKS

18 WEEKS

The fifth month

The bulge caused by the enlarging uterus rises to the level of your navel or just above it, and your weight should be increasing steadily by now.

The baby is still growing rapidly and gaining weight, the foetus is now approximately 24 cm (9½ in.) long and his head is still comparatively large for his body. He can hear sounds from your stomach and rumblings from the bowel. By this month you should have felt your baby kicking and when this happens it's a good idea to make a note of the date just in case there is any confusion over your delivery date.

You will be less sleepy than before and in general should be feeling fit and well – many people think of this stage of pregnancy as the calmest and most pleasant.

The sixth month

It is important that your weight gain should be constant – just under half a kilo (1 lb) a week is ideal. The extra strain may cause some backache but apart from this you will

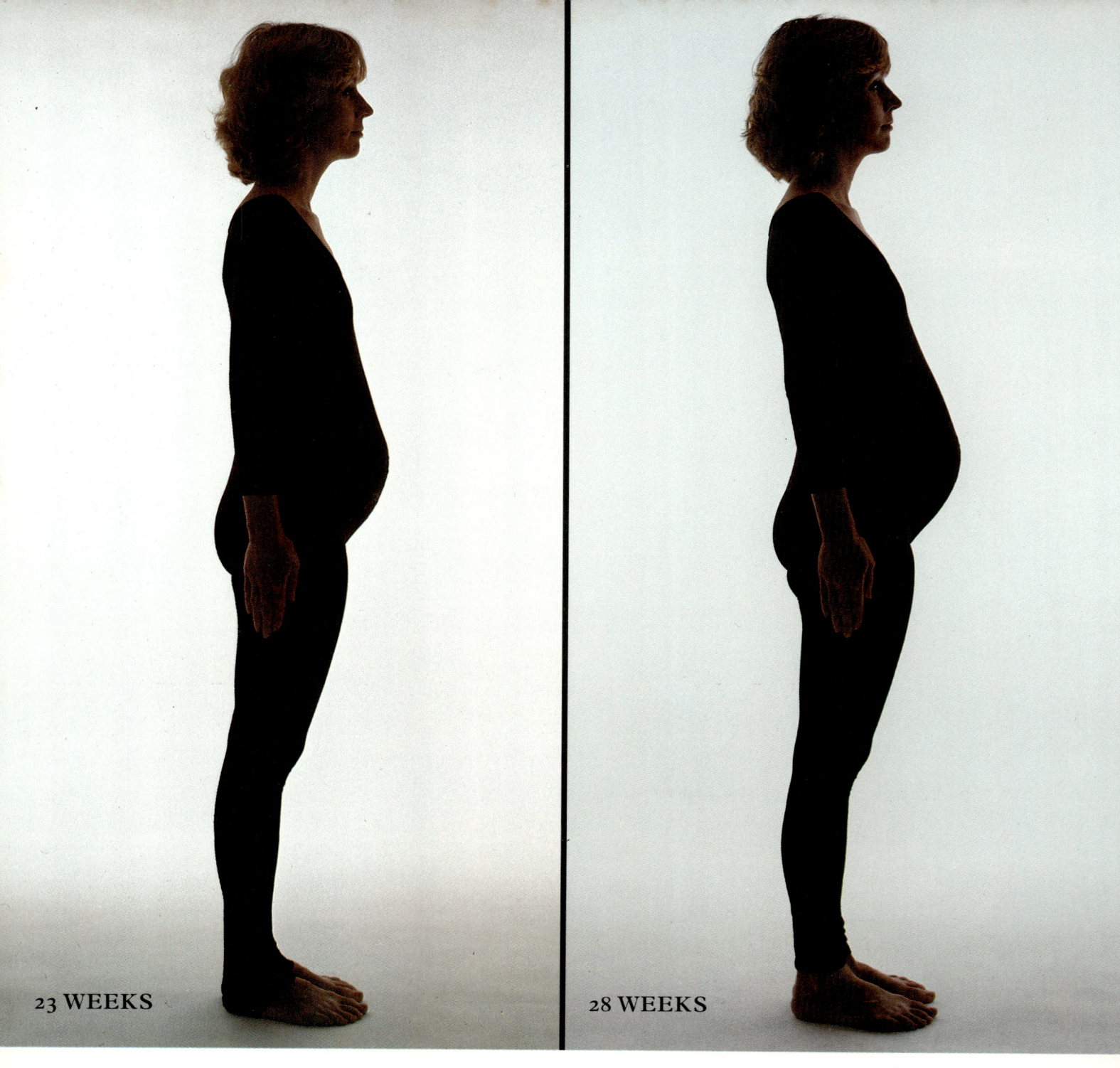

23 WEEKS

28 WEEKS

not feel or look noticeably different to the previous month. Your uterus is still enlarging but the bulge won't look very much bigger.

The baby now weighs about 680 g (1½ lb). He is longer, about 32 cm (12–13 in.), and thin. He has all the organs that he needs for life in the outside world but they are not sufficiently developed to function properly if he were born now. There is also very little fat under the skin and he would not be insulated well enough to keep warm. He would therefore be too premature to survive even in an incubator.

The seventh month

The growing uterus is pushing upwards, squeezing all your organs against your ribcage; you may find it a little difficult to breathe at times and suffer more from heartburn. Your breasts have probably started to secrete colostrum, which is the highly nutritious forerunner to milk. You may find that your appetite has increased and you must be careful not to put on too much weight.

The baby still does not have enough fat for good insulation and if he were born at twenty-eight weeks he would have only

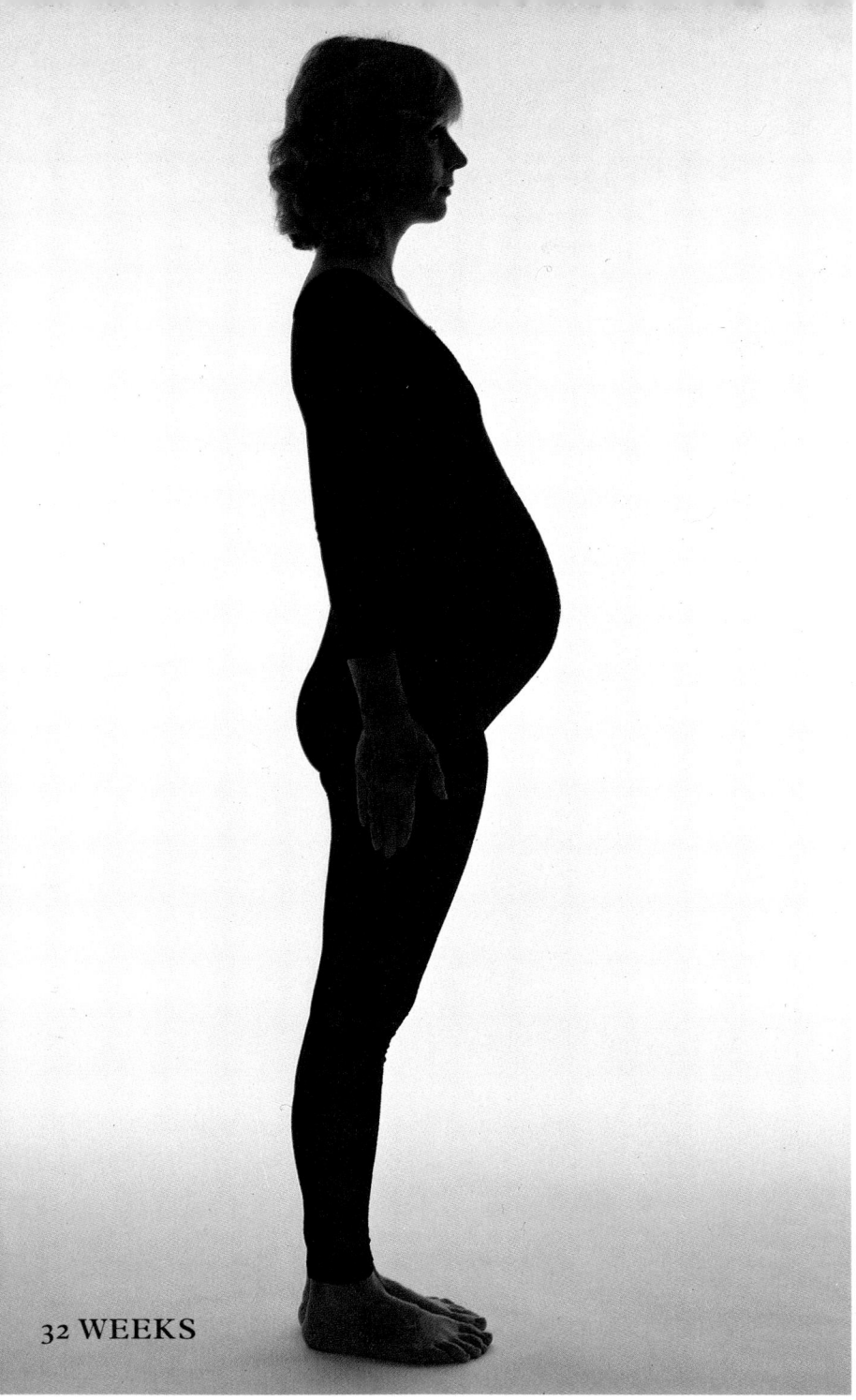

32 WEEKS

may swell noticeably in the evenings. Your 'bump' gets larger as the uterus rises to meet the rib cage. At or around thirty-six weeks the baby's head, which in most cases is pointing downward in readiness for delivery, descends into the pelvis. This is called 'engaging'. As the uterus also drops with it you will find the pressure has been removed from your ribcage making you less prone to heartburn and indigestion. If the head does not descend at this stage there is no cause for concern as this may occur at anytime up to the onset of labour. You may also notice your uterus hardening with 'practice contractions' for delivery. Uterine contractions are a normal phenomenon of pregnancy, which become more regular towards the end of the term. They aid the foetus in that they squeeze out stale blood in the uterus walls, which then refill with fresh blood. These contractions can be distinguished from true labour in that they are not usually painful, are shorter in duration and not as frequent.

The baby's limbs and trunk are growing quite fast now and the body will be in proportion to the head. By the end of the month he will be about 46 cm (18 in.) long and weighs around 2.7 kg (6 lb), having virtually doubled his weight in six weeks. His skin is changing from a reddish colour to a more recognizable pink, as fat begins to be laid down under his skin, and his digestive system is maturing. By the thirty-second week he has a fifteen per cent chance of survival.

The ninth month
You are now in the last weeks of pregnancy and feeling very heavy indeed. The uterus has risen again (having dropped when the baby's head engaged) as the baby puts on a final spurt of growth. He does not move as much as before – the kicking action having given way to squirming and rolling – and will be pressing against your bladder with the result that you will need to pass urine very frequently and find yourself wanting to lean further and further back to counteract the increasing weight in front. Your breasts will be full and heavy, and however tired you feel sleeping may be a problem.

The baby is now fully developed. His length will be about 50 cm (20 in.) long, he weighs about 3.5 kg (7–8 lb) and he has more fat on his body. His organs are able to function and all his reflexes are working; he has fingernails and hair, he can see, hear and smell, and his lungs and voice are ready to go into action the minute he takes his first gulp of air.

about a five per cent chance of survival, if he were healthy. He is about 2.5 cm (1 in.) longer and weighs 55–85 g (2–3 lb) and is now filling a lot of the space in the uterus. Whereas before he was swimming and kicking freely in the amniotic fluid of the womb he will soon be finding it difficult to turn himself round. His behaviour is beginning to form a pattern. It is not known whether babies actually sleep in the uterus but they have periods of activity and quiet.

The eighth month
You will be feeling more and more sluggish as this month progresses and your ankles

You and Your Emotions

While everyone expects you to be happy, radiant and content as a mother-to-be, there may well be times when you feel depressed, anxious, irritable, even suddenly and inexplicably in tears, no matter how delighted you are with yourself and your growing baby. Such down-in-the-dumps feelings can last five minutes, or might continue all day, but usually they disappear as suddenly as they arrived. Anything may set you off; a chance remark about your looks or mood, or any one of the little things that can go wrong at home. Your forgetfulness, overwhelming tiredness and sudden anxieties about the future can all depress you. But while you and all those around you should be prepared for some uncharacteristic changes of mood, you don't have any excuse to be permanently bad-tempered. It's unlikely that you will feel depressed for any length of time – but if you do don't be afraid to seek medical advice.

Women commonly experience emotional 'lows' during puberty, the menopause and just before a period, due to the rising and falling of hormone levels in the body. Some women taking the birth control pill report similar reactions from time to time. Similarly, in pregnancy the exceptionally rapid increase of certain hormones, particularly the major female hormones oestrogen and progesterone, can be emotionally unsettling. Progesterone, especially, is produced in large quantities at the onset of pregnancy and is the cause of the earlier symptoms, notably the enlargement of the breasts and sensations of nausea during the first weeks.

During the first three months of pregnancy your body is going through its most drastic upheaval – a single fertilized cell is growing minute by minute into a human being. By the end of twelve weeks your baby will be fully formed and swimming in the fluid around him. All that has to happen now is for him to mature, develop and grow bigger and stronger. Once this initial phenomenon has happened hormone levels settle down, and as nausea and tiredness recede and your appetite returns, together with the blooming good looks characteristic of pregnant women, you should find that you feel emotionally more settled too. Irritability, outbursts of temper and sudden emotional changes from high to low and back should be much less frequent.

Your circumstances as well as the physical changes may affect the way you feel. If the pregnancy is unexpected or unwanted, and you have had to make a difficult decision to go ahead and have the child, you will almost certainly experience sharp fluctuations of mood. Looking after

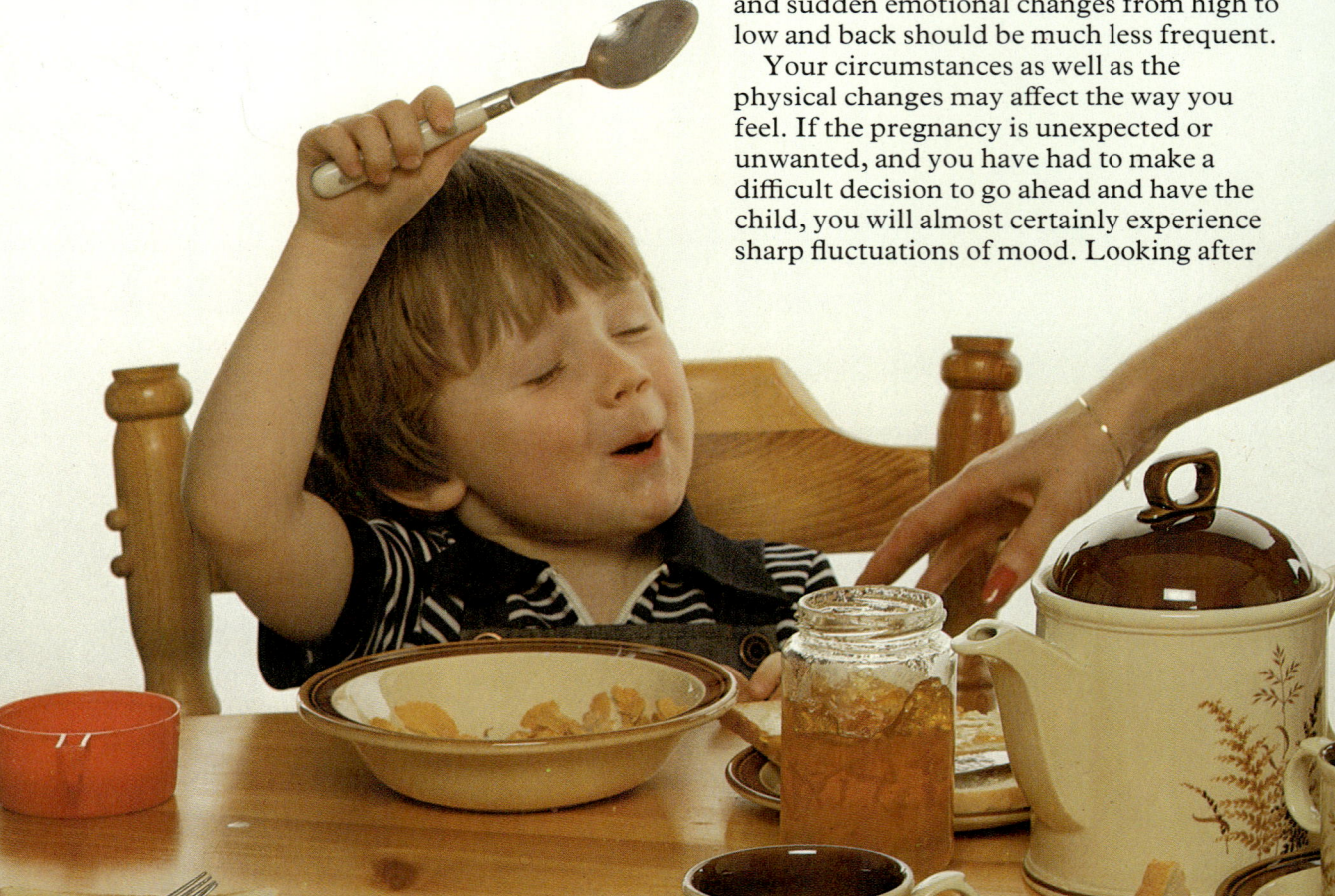

small children can make you feel emotionally drained especially if you are suffering from nausea and sickness during the first fourteen weeks. If the sickness really gets you down, your doctor should be able to prescribe a safe anti-nausea remedy.

Understanding from those around you is a definite bonus – of course you need sympathy and comfort – but at the same time you don't want an overdose of indulgence. Everyone has bad days and even though you may feel especially sensitive, try not to fall into a morass of self pity. Don't neglect yourself or remain cooped up at home brooding, instead make an effort to get out and seek the company of others you can talk to – friends with small children have been through it all before and can be of invaluable help.

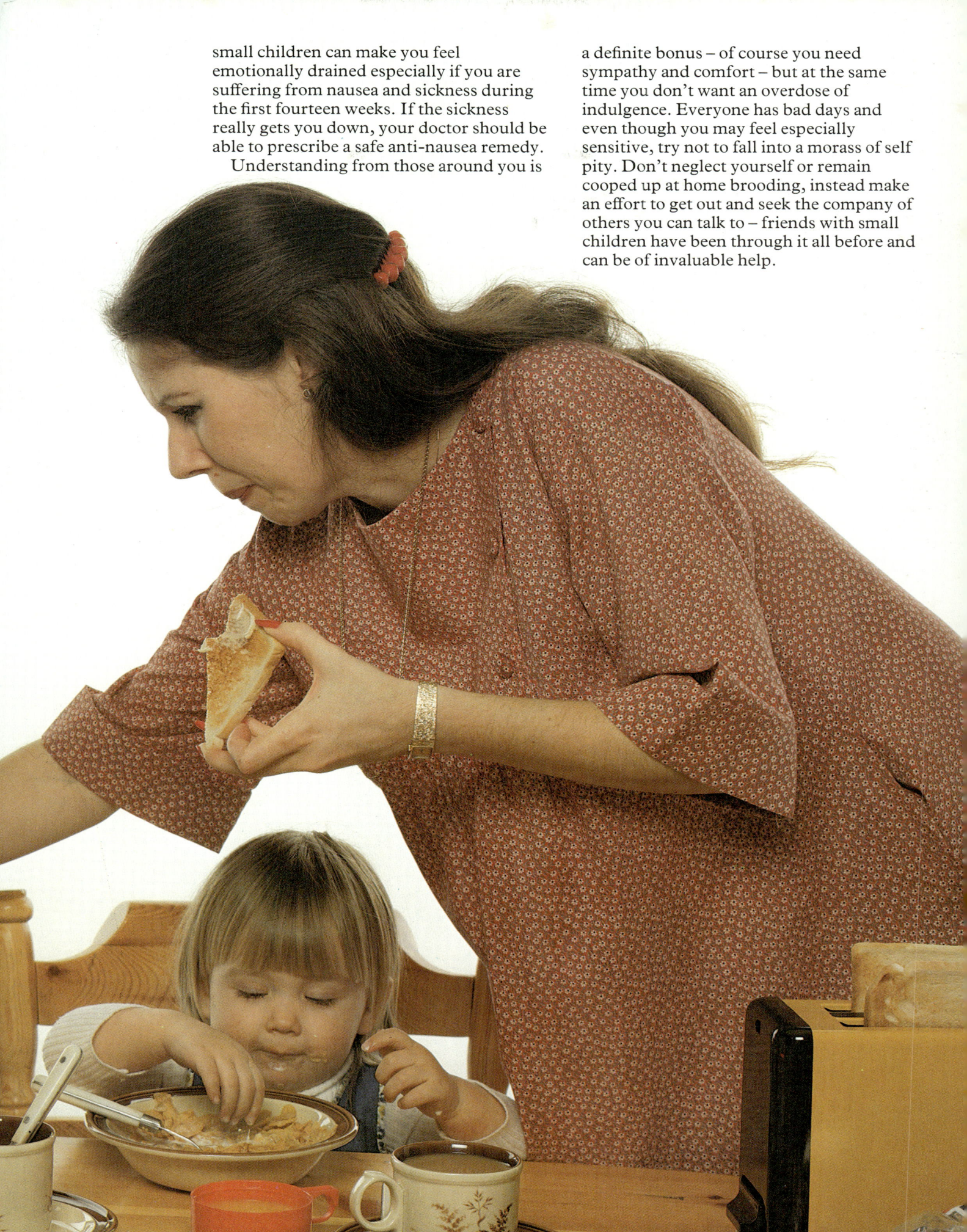

One of those days

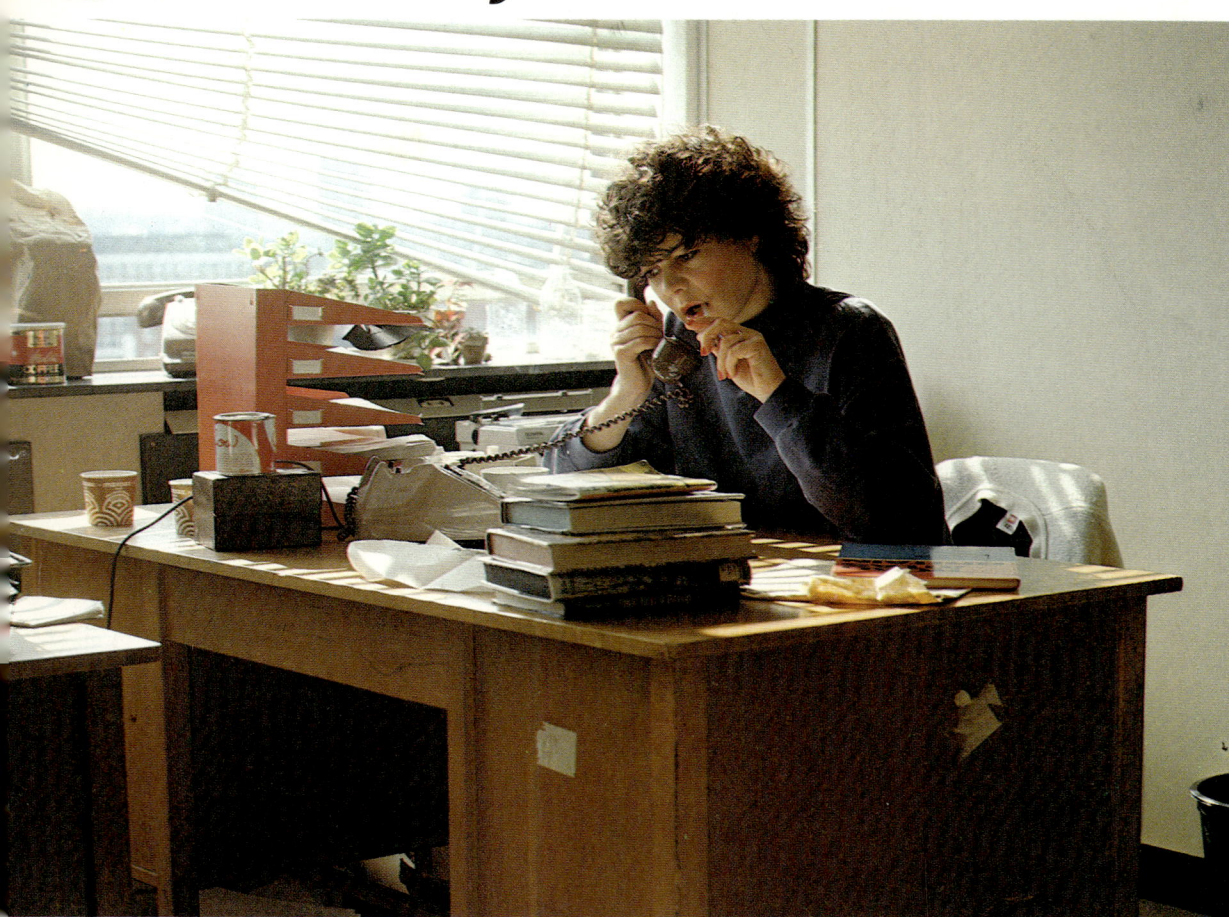

We've found that a pregnant woman is likely to experience at least one really memorable black day, when the morning starts badly and the rest of the day is just a downward spiral as you become increasingly emotional and overwrought. At work phones ring and problems have to be dealt with, but today you just can't cope with the busy office routine as well as you would normally.

Does your mood affect your baby?

You will probably hear many old wives tales during your pregnancy, most of which you can safely ignore. Certainly stories that strange sights or nightmares can adversely affect an unborn child through his mother's reaction are simply rubbish, and you can dismiss them from your thoughts. It's unlikely that your general state of mind will be transferred to your baby and day-to-day anxieties will not harm him. It is known, however, that in pregnancy the baby in the uterus reacts to physical influences from the outside world. In later pregnancy, he can hear loud noises like a bang in the room and can even notice strong light from the outside world penetrating his mother's abdomen. You may notice that your baby starts kicking jerkily if you are particularly agitated so obviously the more relaxed you are, the better for both of you, and try not to subject him to sudden physical shocks. Fortunately many pregnant women find that they become increasingly contented.

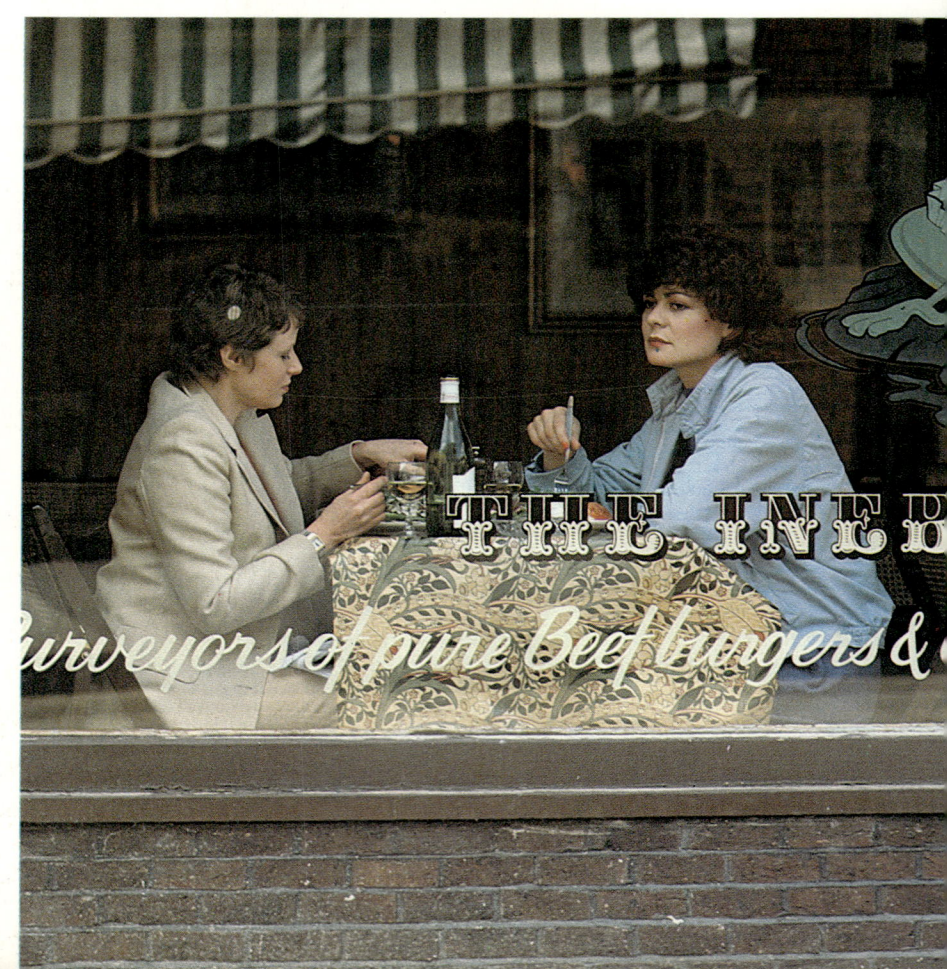

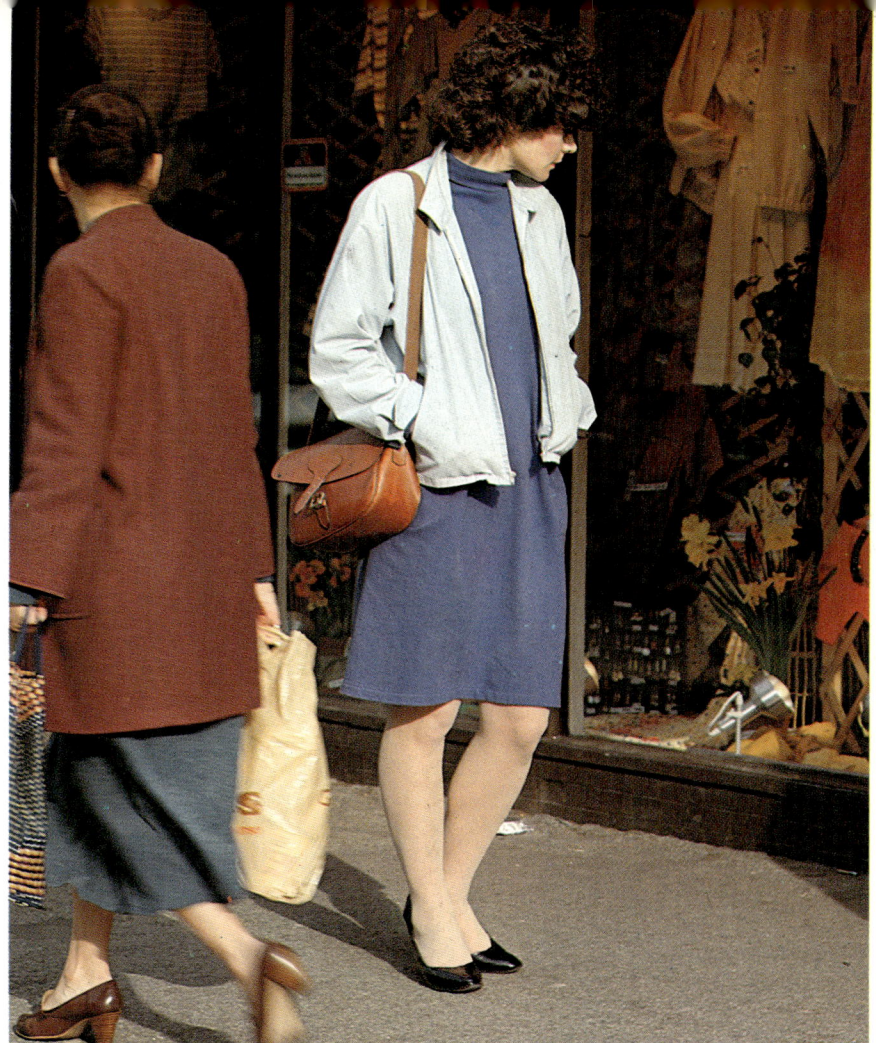

5.30

You decide to go late-night shopping to cheer yourself up but today even this turns out to be a depressing business. All fashions seem to be designed for rakes not expectant mothers and you feel ever more dowdy in your enlarging smock. Finally you find a dress to try on, only to be exasperated when the wraith-like assistant suggests that perhaps it would look better nipped in at the waist with a belt!

6.30

You arrive home exhausted and tearful and convinced you are never going to enjoy life again. Pregnancy is supposed to be a wonderful experience, but today you've just felt tired, unattractive and thoroughly left out of things. Don't despair, ring up any friend who has had a baby and you'll probably find that she can recount a similar tale of woe – and comfort yourself that though today has been awful, tomorrow will certainly be better.

12.30

You meet a non-pregnant friend for lunch, but the smell of cooking suddenly puts you off your food and she looks smarter than you feel and enviably thin. People can sometimes be unwittingly tactless in their reaction to your pregnancy and today you are terribly oversensitive to well-worn jokes and thoughtless remarks, especially about your increasing size.

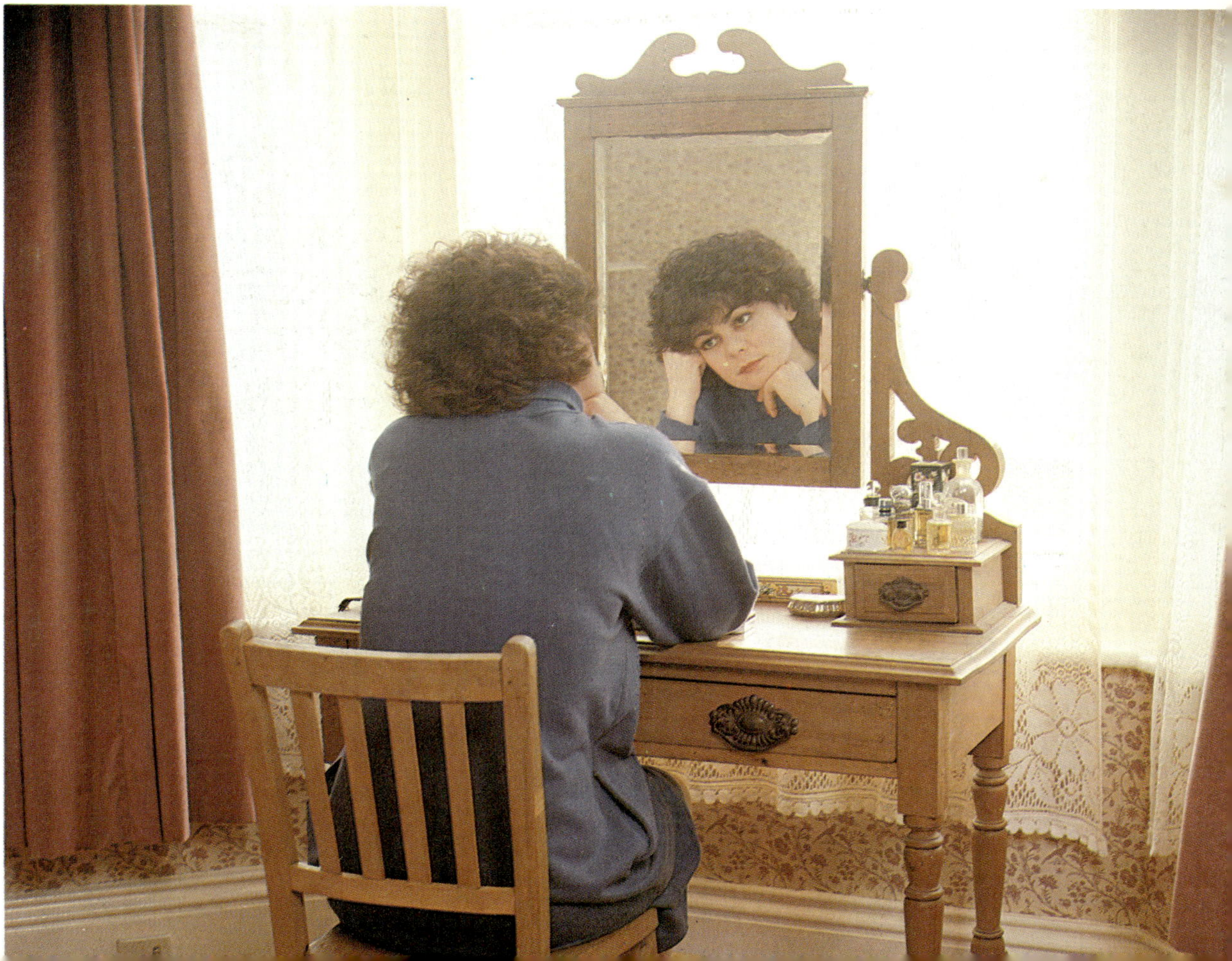

Coping with tiredness

An overwhelming tiredness accompanied by apathy and lassitude is usual during early pregnancy and you will find you need a lot of rest at this time. But together with morning sickness the exhaustion should pass after fourteen weeks, to be replaced by revived energy and a sense of well-being that will give you a new bloom and sparkle. Inevitably the tiredness will start to catch up with you again in the last three months as your body has more and more weight to carry around, and by the final weeks you will have to accept that you simply can't do everything you would like.

The best way to cope with tiredness is not to fight it. If you feel like a catnap – which is usually all you need in the middle of the day – give in. The ideal amount of rest is ten hours in every twenty-four. This could be eight hours sleep at night and two hours rest or sleep during the day, although it's impossible to be specific about how many hours of sleep each person needs. Try to get a good eight to ten hours in bed at night even if you are reading or listening to the radio some of the time. Cancel arrangements if you don't feel like going out. You will only get more tired and irritable if you don't take heed of what your body is telling you. If you already have children you may feel more tired than in your first pregnancy and obviously you will find it difficult to fit in an afternoon rest. Take any opportunity to sit down and relax and when you do always put your feet up. Ask friends or neighbours to look after your children for an hour or two each day to give you a break, or consider enrolling them at a nursery or playgroup if there is one in your area to which they could go.

Being at work presents difficulties in finding time to relax, too. In this case it's a good idea to sit quietly with your legs up

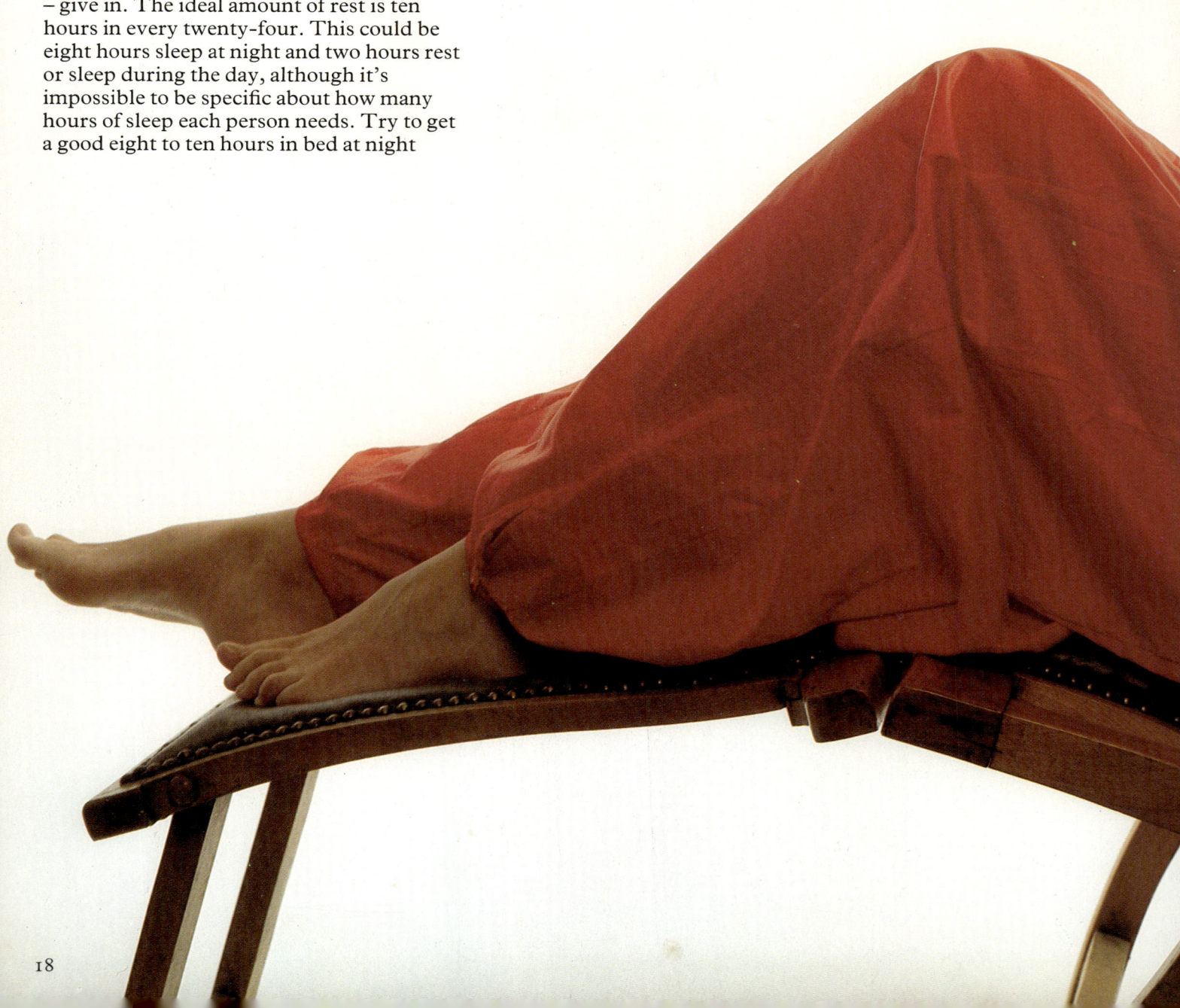

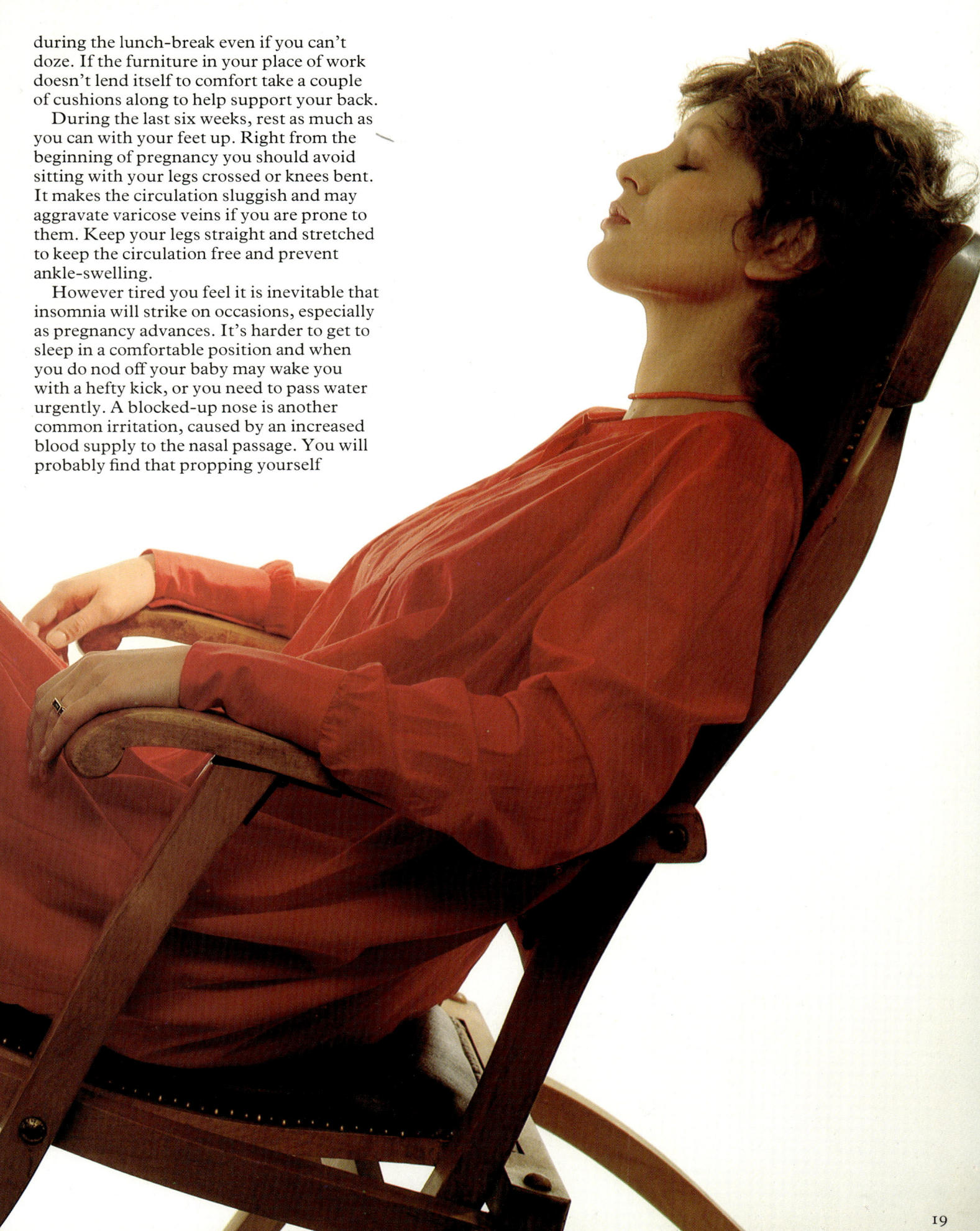

during the lunch-break even if you can't doze. If the furniture in your place of work doesn't lend itself to comfort take a couple of cushions along to help support your back.

During the last six weeks, rest as much as you can with your feet up. Right from the beginning of pregnancy you should avoid sitting with your legs crossed or knees bent. It makes the circulation sluggish and may aggravate varicose veins if you are prone to them. Keep your legs straight and stretched to keep the circulation free and prevent ankle-swelling.

However tired you feel it is inevitable that insomnia will strike on occasions, especially as pregnancy advances. It's harder to get to sleep in a comfortable position and when you do nod off your baby may wake you with a hefty kick, or you need to pass water urgently. A blocked-up nose is another common irritation, caused by an increased blood supply to the nasal passage. You will probably find that propping yourself upright with some extra pillows is a comfortable position or that lying on your side with a pillow under your abdomen is a good way to prevent the uterus literally dragging you over. A firm bed is always an advantage especially if you suffer from backache. If your mattress is soft, place some wooden boards underneath it, or a large sheet of hardboard with holes drilled in it to let the mattress 'breathe'.

The calmer your mind is, the more relaxed your body will be. So do try and banish the worries of the day – the old tip of counting sheep can be helpful. Let every muscle in your body go limp . . . let your jaw sag . . . loosen your facial muscles. Breathe slowly in through your nose and out through your mouth – not too deeply or you will feel dizzy from the intake of too much oxygen. Whatever you do, don't worry about not sleeping; the more worried you become that you can't sleep, the more elusive sleep will be. Lack of sleep does not affect your physical health, and it will not raise your blood pressure.

Your doctor will not prescribe sleeping pills in early pregnancy, but during the last few months there are some particularly mild ones that he may be happy for you to take. A hot, milky drink just before bedtime is often sleep-inducing or you might find that herbal remedies such as camomile tea are helpful. Ask advice at a local health shop. A good night's sleep certainly makes a difference to the way you look as well as the way you feel. Tiredness aggravates puffy eyes whereas a good night's sleep helps to make them look bright and the whites whiter.

Keep your interests going

'In the club' is an apt expression for pregnancy; your thoughts are naturally focussed on yourself and your changing body and you tend to gravitate towards others in the same condition to exchange notes. Lasting friendships are often formed at antenatal clinics or mothercraft classes based on the one overwhelming, all-consuming interest you are sharing. There is nothing wrong in that, but don't exclude your family and non-pregnant friends from your thoughts and conversation. You will need to tread a fine line between involving them in your experience on the one hand and boring them rigid on the other.

Never allow pregnancy to take over your life completely. Having outside interests is a definite help. If you are working and have an absorbing job, so much the better.

Unless you find it becomes too physically taxing there is no reason why you should not carry on working until the last six weeks or so.

If you are a career woman and have to give up work and financial independence earlier than you had planned, it is understandable that you might find it hard to come to terms with your new life. Having enjoyed a fulfilling job you may well resent the fact that you are going to be out of the action for some time and the sudden drop in income is bound to be tough. Make sure that you have applied for all the maternity benefits you are entitled to (see page 75) and make plans for your return to work after the baby is born. Meanwhile keep your existing interests going if practicable, or make the most of the opportunity and take up a new hobby or the evening class you never had time for before. You will almost certainly find something going on in your area to interest you. Your local library will be able to give you information on what's going on and where.

(see page 75)

Right: Place a cushion or pillow behind the small of your back when resting, if the chair doesn't properly support your spine. Remember to sit with your legs straight rather than crossed to avoid varicose veins, and put your feet up whenever you can – they should be level with your bottom or higher.

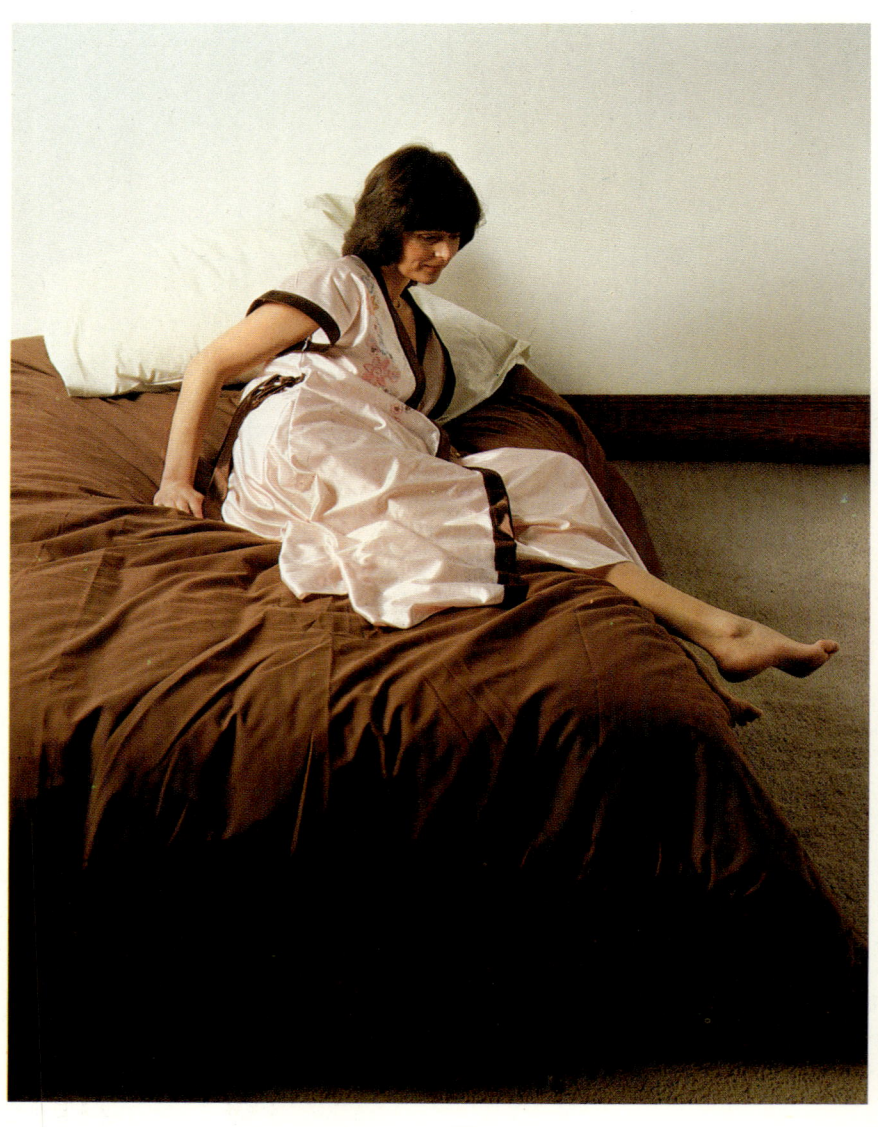

20

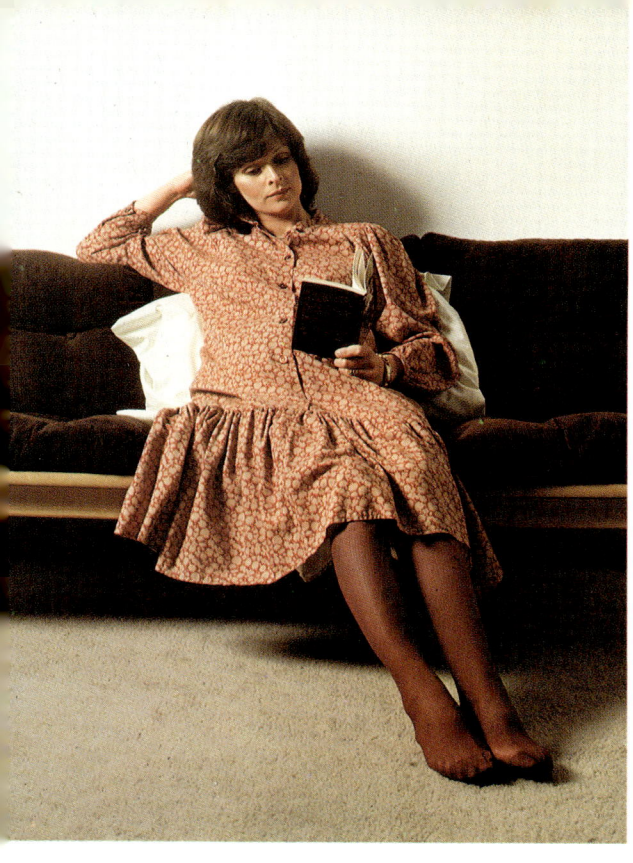

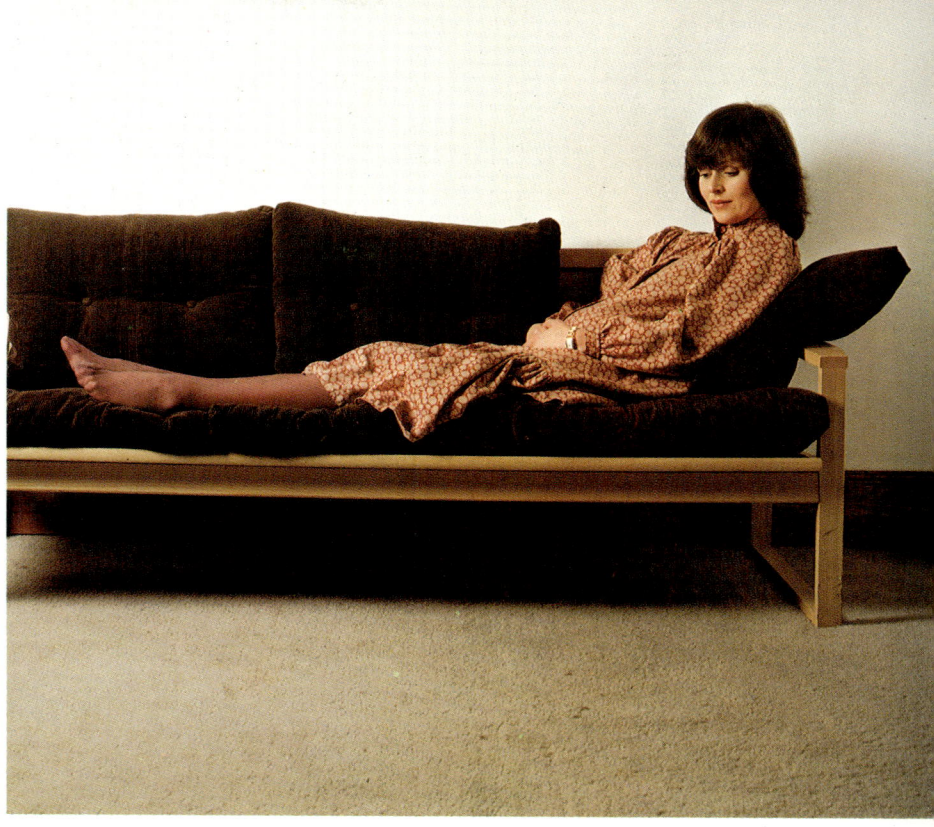

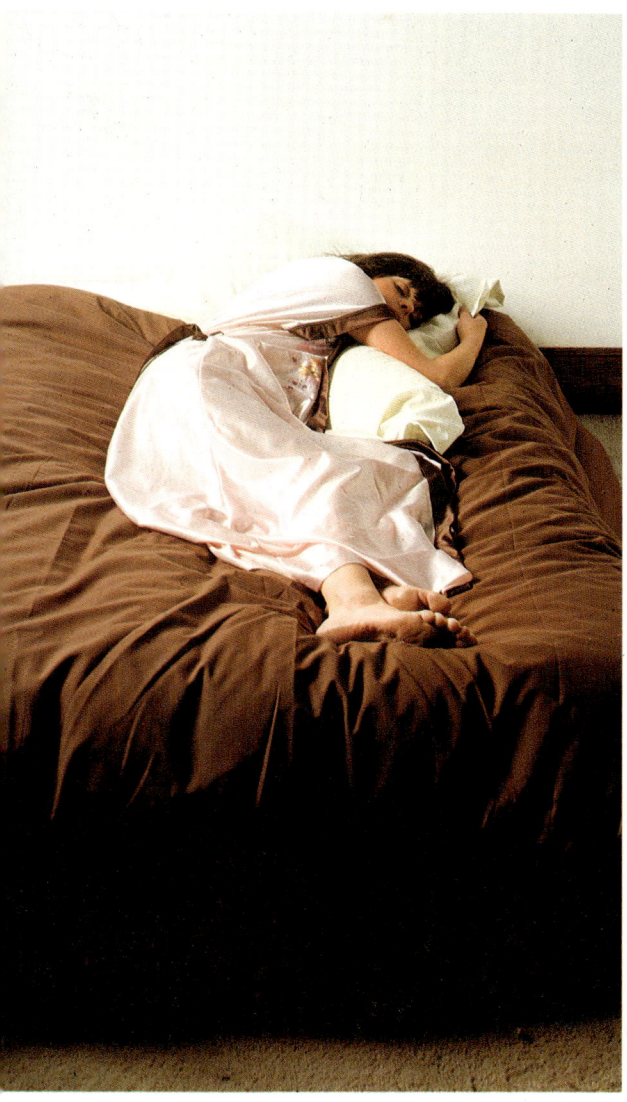

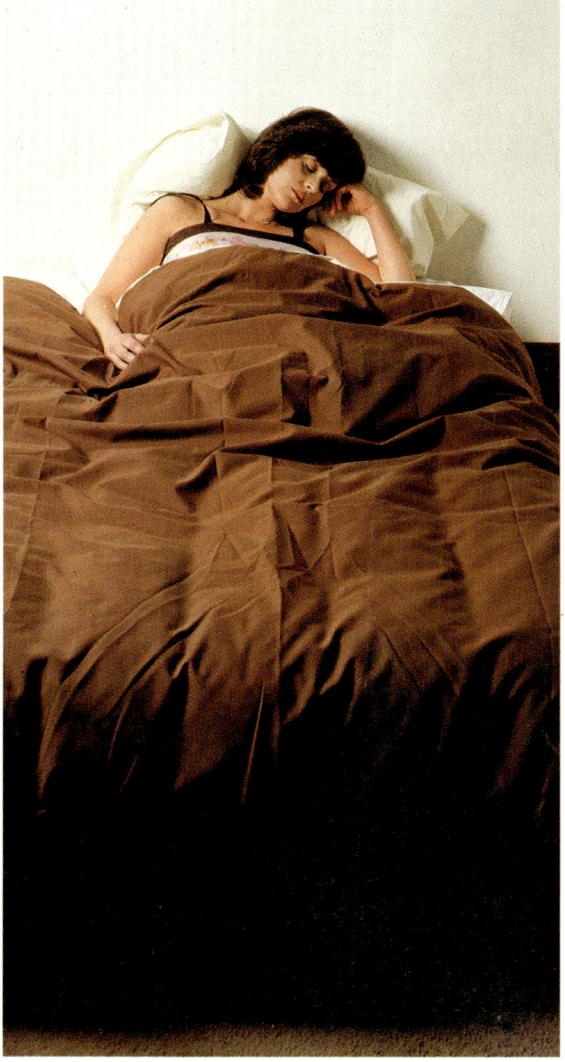

Far left: Don't leap out of bed too quickly in the morning, just in case you feel giddy, and never pull yourself up by your stomach muscles. Roll on to one side first and push yourself up on your elbow before swinging your legs over the side.

Left: Finding a comfortable sleeping position becomes more difficult as pregnancy advances. Lying on your side with the abdomen supported by a pillow is probably the most effective way to get to sleep. If you suffer from heartburn, try propping yourself in a sitting position.

Lovemaking

You and your partner should feel especially close at this time in your lives, yet some pregnant women do quite genuinely 'go off' sex. They may find it distasteful, think it might harm the baby, or just become bored.

It is perfectly possible to enjoy lovemaking during pregnancy, providing you have no history of miscarriage. However, if you are prone to miscarriage, any strong activity during the early months could affect the blood circulation and so disturb the pregnancy. Thus if you have previously lost a baby your doctor may advise against intercourse during the first fourteen weeks. (For the same reason, he will probably not perform an internal examination during this time.) In a few cases – for example if an ultrasound scan shows the placenta to be lying low in the uterus – he might advise total abstinence until the baby is born.

As you become more ungainly you could feel concerned that your partner finds you less sexually attractive in your pregnant state. There is no reason why he should. For while it is true that some men do find pregnancy off-putting, many men appreciate the added curves and continue to find their partners just as desirable – if not more so. It is up to him just as much as to you to show that nothing has changed. Talk over how you feel, and both try to come to terms with your changing body. After all, it won't be like that for ever.

Many women, in fact, enjoy their sex life more than ever during pregnancy, finding it fulfilling and satisfying. They discover that it is easy to carry on lovemaking throughout pregnancy by adopting positions to suit the increasing discomfort of the growing abdomen. As in everything, patience and

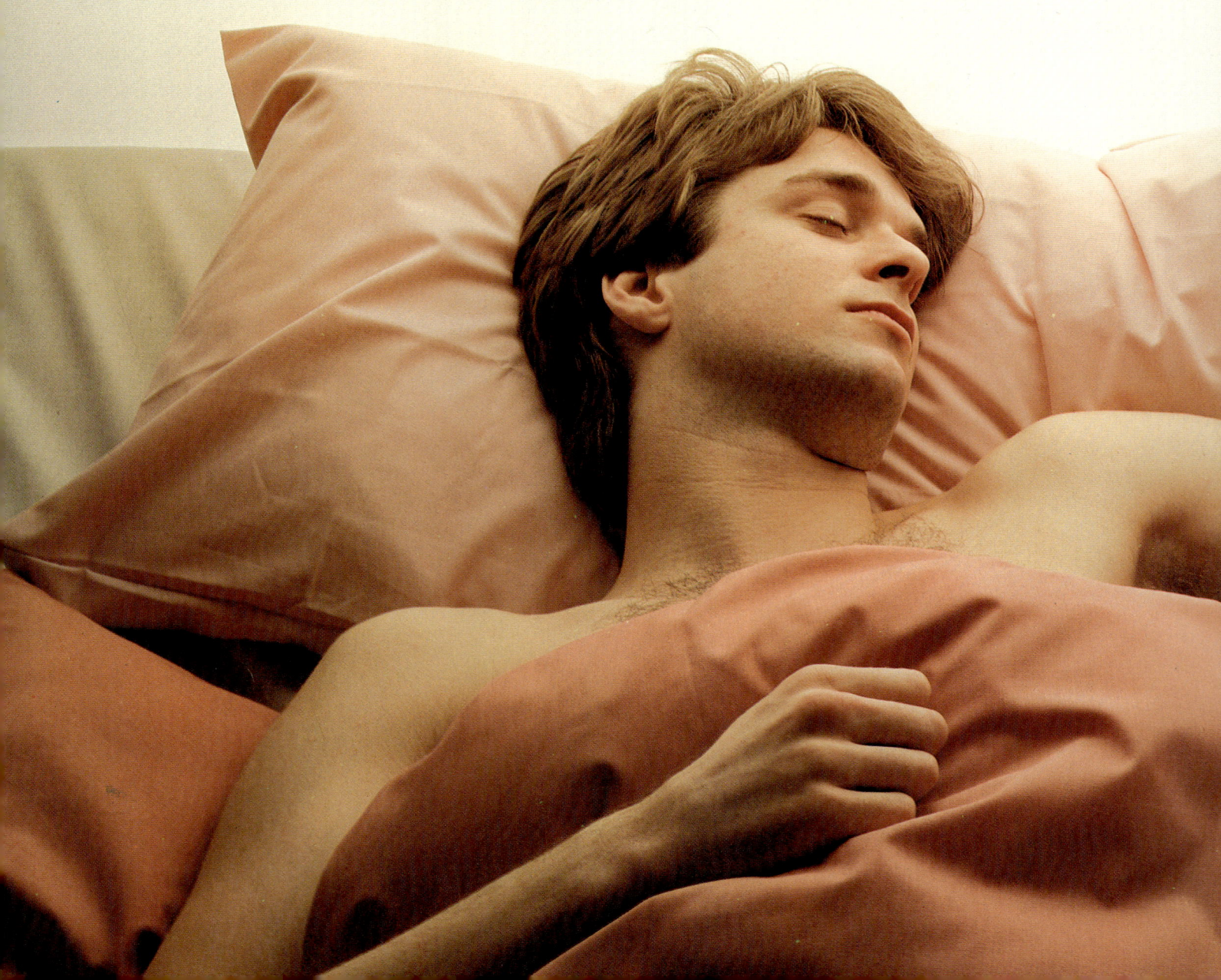

understanding on both sides is always important.

Towards the end of your pregnancy there is a possibility that lovemaking could initiate labour if the baby is ready to be born. Intercourse itself cannot harm the baby, but your orgasm might set off contractions of the uterus strong enough to cause you to go into labour. It is often suggested that the hormone prostaglandin found in the male semen may bring on labour, since this same hormone is used in pessaries that are given to help induce labour artificially. However, the amount of prostaglandin found in the semen is such a minute quantity that this can be discounted as exceptionally unlikely. While it is as well to be aware that intercourse could speed up the course of events, doctors will not generally advise you to stop. A woman's libido, anyway, will decline naturally towards the impending birth.

The first kick

The highs of pregnancy tend to far outweigh the lows. Carrying a child is a miraculous work of nature however ungainly, bumbling and even downright miserable you feel at times. Feeling the baby move for the first time can be a thrilling moment. This is usually between the twentieth and the twenty-second week in a first pregnancy, but can be as early as the fourteenth week in a subsequent one – the average time is around the eighteenth week. If you have never experienced that first 'flutter' it won't be anything like you've imagined, even though friends will graphically describe 'air bubbles popping', 'butterflies', even 'wind'. It will be all these things yet none of them, but however you yourself identify this first real sign of life, it's a comforting and emotional time.

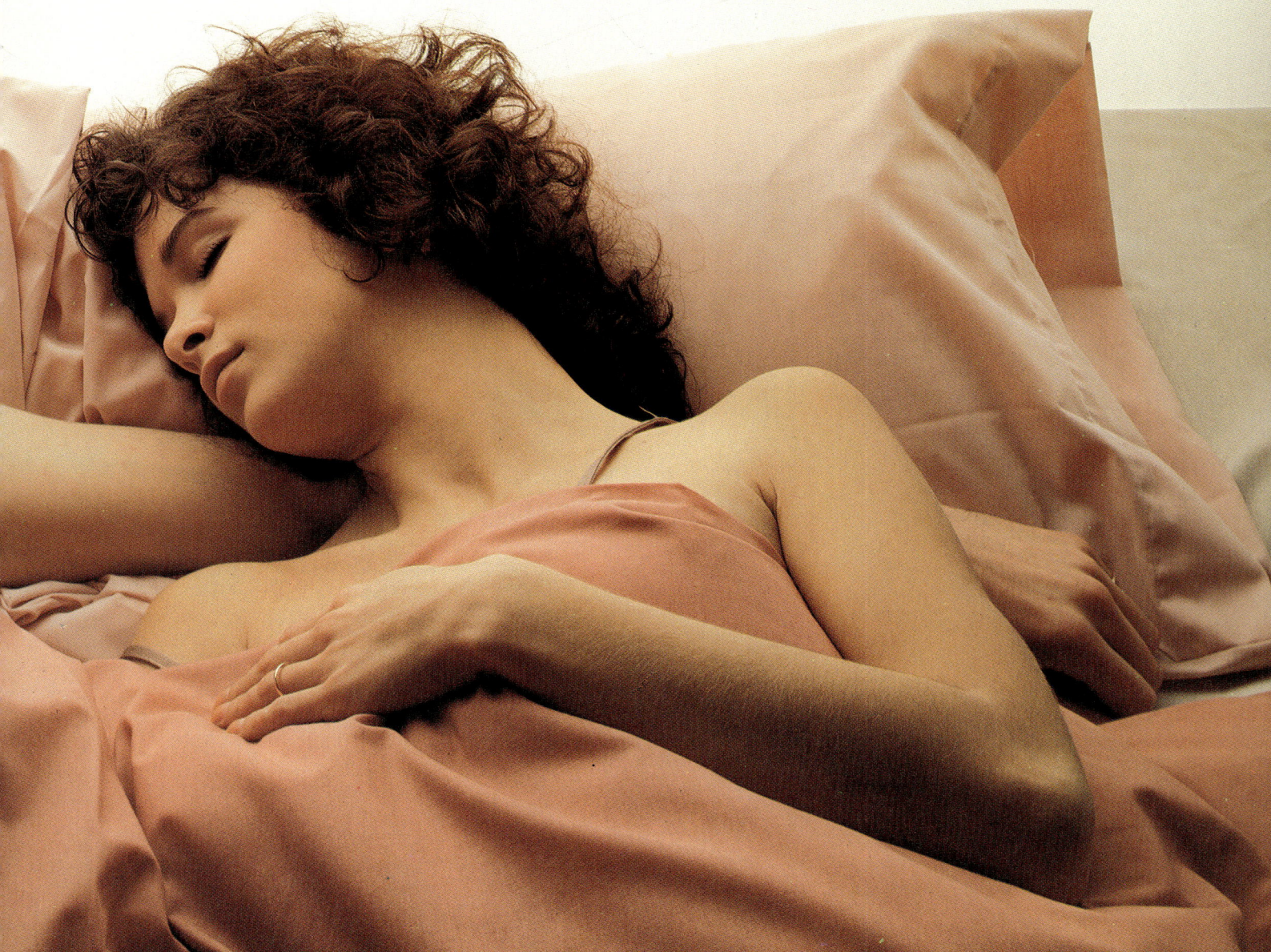

Body Care

Your skin and muscles are stretched quite radically during pregnancy and labour, and if you allow yourself to become out of condition may take some time to return to normal afterwards. A little care and regular exercise can do a lot towards keeping you fit and supple while you are pregnant, and help to restore your figure after the birth.

Pregnancy inevitably brings about all kinds of minor changes to the body apart from the obvious bulge. The important thing is not to worry about these, but to understand what is happening and why. Every woman and every pregnancy is totally different and you may sail through your pregnancy with little or no inconvenient side effects. However, it is just as well to be aware of what changes can happen so that you know how to cope with them should they arise.

Breasts

The breasts do not contain muscle and once they are allowed to sag no amount of exercise will ever revive them. So a good supporting bra as you enlarge during pregnancy is absolutely essential.

You should make sure that your breasts are firmly supported at about the tenth week, by which time they will probably be noticeably larger. Check their size again at the twentieth week – often there is another noticeable increase by this stage. Your breasts should then remain the same size until delivery, but make sure that your bra has several alteration hooks at the back as the chest wall expands by an inch or two towards the end of pregnancy due to the ligaments relaxing.

For a lot of women, the improved bust that pregnancy brings is a welcome bonus and a look at some of the bulky, unflattering maternity bras available could well be depressing. Don't despair – there are plenty of pretty, fashionable bras on the market that will give you perfectly adequate support. As long as the bra has strong, fairly wide shoulder straps (narrow elastic is not sufficiently supportive), good uplift underneath and a wide adjustable back, you can choose anything from fresh broderie anglaise to sexy black lace. If you find that your breasts feel heavy at night a light unribbed sleeping bra may be advisable.

To find your correct size, measure directly under the bust next to the skin and round this figure up to the nearest standard bra size. To get the correct cup size – which is the measurement most likely to increase – measure the fullest part of the bust and shoulder blades. If the difference between the two measurements you have taken is under 15 cm (6 in.) then you need a B cup; if it is over 15 cm (6 in.) you want a C cup; and if even greater, try a D cup.

Don't buy a nursing bra – that is one that opens at the front to enable you to breastfeed – until the last month of pregnancy when you have a good idea of the size your breasts will be after the birth. Again, make sure the bra you choose has adjustable hooks at the back to cope with changes in breast size after the milk arrives.

Wash your breasts daily when you take your regular bath or shower, but be sparing with the soap as this can be drying. To keep the nipples supple in preparation for breastfeeding, massage them gently every day with a little oil, lanolin or nipple cream.

Abdomen

If you have never worn a girdle and haven't put on an excessive amount of weight there is really no need to wear one now – with care and exercise your muscles will return to normal soon after you have had your baby. However, some women do find that mid-way through pregnancy they have a certain amount of aching in the lower abdomen; a feeling of dragging down. If you feel this kind of muscular discomfort or your abdomen becomes very large, a lightweight maternity girdle will help. If you normally wear a girdle then, of course, you must not discard it during pregnancy as your muscles will not be able to cope. As long as it is still comfortable, wear your normal girdle, which will stretch as you get bigger, or buy a maternity girdle, which gives particular support to the lower abdominal muscles. When you find you are growing out of a girdle, replace it with another straight away – don't give the muscles a chance to sag. It's an old wives' tale that support underwear can damage the baby in the uterus – so don't fear that you may be squashing him; he's well protected by the thick walls of the womb. It's your own comfort that's the important thing here. When choosing a girdle, always measure the widest part of the hips, about 20 cm (8 in.) below the waist.

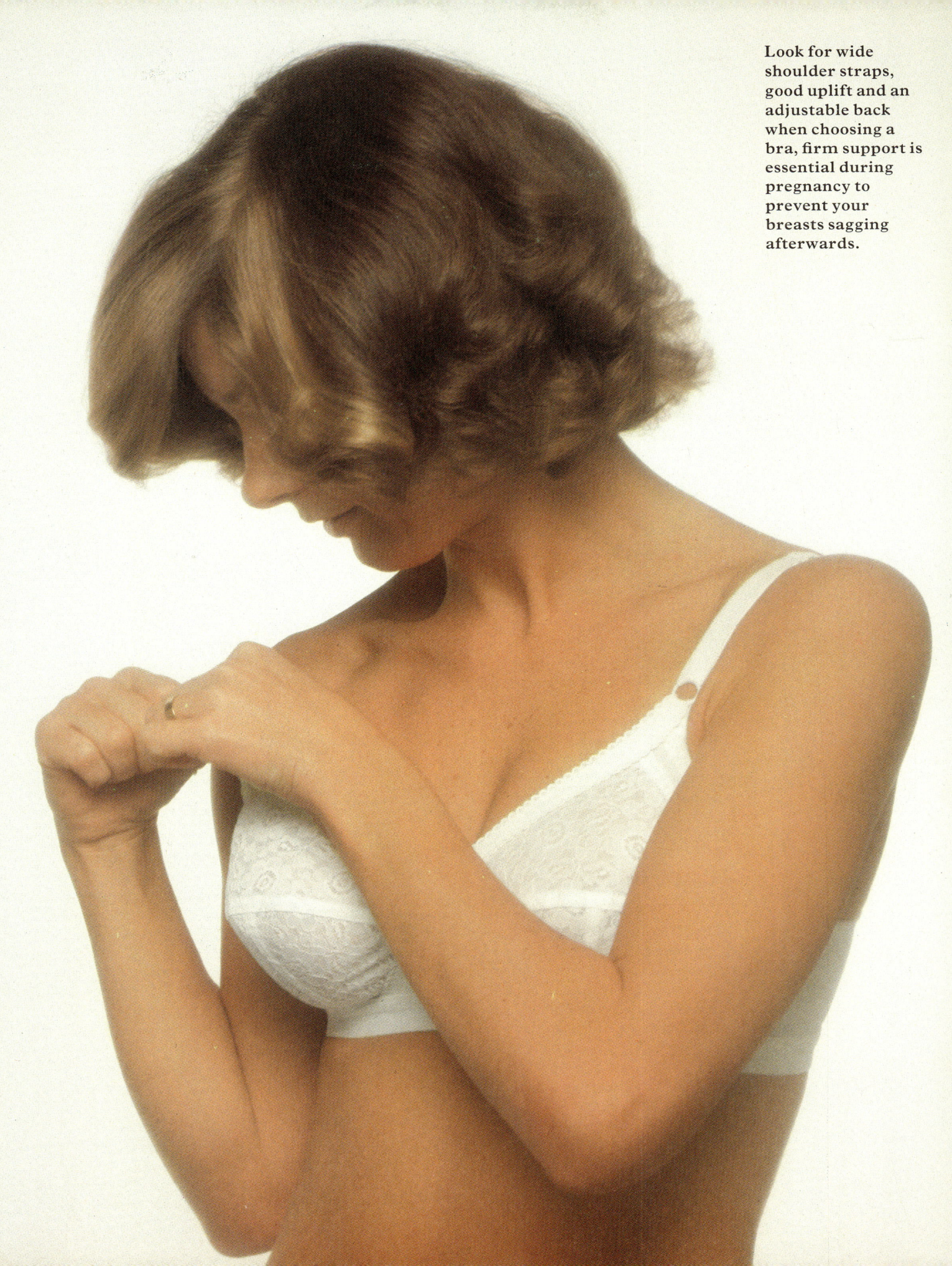

Look for wide shoulder straps, good uplift and an adjustable back when choosing a bra, firm support is essential during pregnancy to prevent your breasts sagging afterwards.

Backache and posture

The best way to prevent backache is to make sure that your posture is correct. The hormone progesterone causes the tendons and ligaments of the body to soften and stretch, especially in the back and pelvis, and the strain caused by the weight of the baby on the lower joints of the spine can cause a nagging, uncomfortable ache. A firm bed, massage and an electric pad or a hot water bottle wrapped in a cover and placed on the back will all help, but if you stand as upright as possible and avoid the pregnancy slouch (the classic droop of the shoulders and relaxation of the stomach) you will improve your posture and be less prone to backache. To check your posture, stand with your back against a wall, balance your weight evenly between the balls and heels of your feet, pull your abdomen in and make yourself as tall as possible. Try and keep this straight stance whether standing still or walking.

Strain on the back can of course be caused by bending or lifting badly. When you pick anything up, always bend your knees and keep your back straight. Never try bending from the waist, which will pull the muscles in your back. Remember this when picking up a small child or pet. If you have a lot of shopping to carry, never pile it all into one bag, spread the load evenly between two bags and carry one in each hand. But don't attempt to carry more than you can comfortably manage.

Housework can also cause posture problems. Try to sit at the sink or ironing board rather than stand; kneel to make the bed rather than bend; kneel by the side of the bath to clean it.

The pelvic floor

The softening of the joints and ligaments during pregnancy is necessary because the pelvis needs to be as flexible as possible for the birth. For the same reason it is important to keep the pelvic floor – the large muscle that supports your pelvic organs – toned up in preparation for labour. If you practise these simple exercises now, they will also help after your baby is born in getting your muscles back into shape.

1 Tighten and relax the ring of muscles immediately around the anus (back passage), keeping your stomach and buttock muscles relaxed.

2 Tense and relax the muscles that surround openings of the bladder and vagina – as if stopping yourself passing urine. In fact, this is a good time to practise pelvic floor exercises – a few minutes stream-stopping every day will do a lot towards toning you up.

3 Now pull up the whole of the pelvic floor by contracting both sets of muscles together. You can do these exercises anywhere – while driving the car, standing at the bus stop – whenever you have a spare minute and remember.

Stretch marks

Stretch marks are thin red scar-like lines that appear very suddenly during pregnancy where the skin stretches on the abdomen, breasts, or thighs. After the birth they gradually fade to silvery marks, but never disappear completely. Some women seem to be more prone to them than others and are likely to get them if they put on too much weight. Apart from watching your weight gain there is no way of preventing stretch marks and creaming or oiling the skin with exorbitantly priced 'wonder preparations' will not be effective. However as the skin often becomes dry during pregnancy creaming will certainly help to keep it supple. Antenatal cream, vitamin E oil or a little baby oil in the bath will all make your skin feel softer.

Pigmentation and sunbathing

There is usually an increase in pigmentation of the skin during pregnancy, which brunettes find most noticeable – freckles, birth-marks, moles and some scars seem to get much darker, especially if they are exposed to the sun. The nipples and areola – the area of delicate skin around the nipple – change colour at around the fourteenth week of pregnancy either changing from pink to brown or simply becoming darker. Again, this is far more marked in dark-haired women than in women with fair skin who have very little pigmentation of the breasts. A dark line called the *linea nigra* develops down the middle of the abdomen at about the same time. The line can stretch from the pubic hair to the lower ribs, but often only extends as far as the umbilicus (which can also pigment and flatten towards the end of pregnancy). It usually

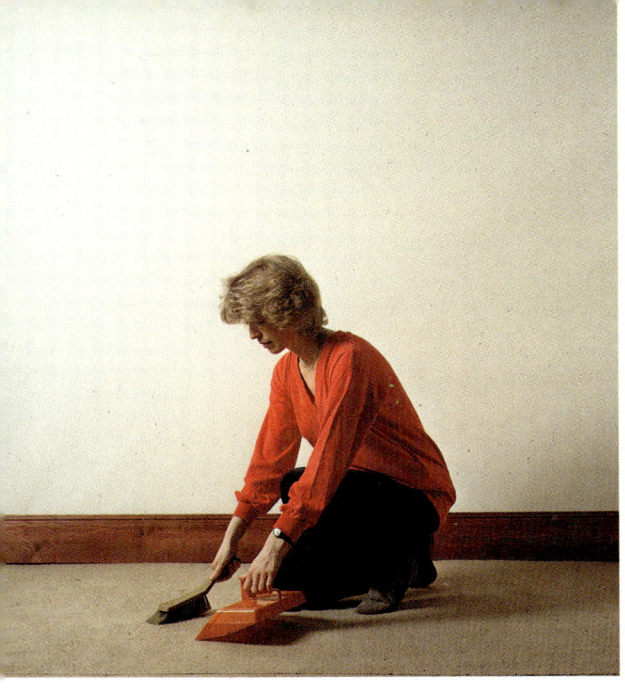

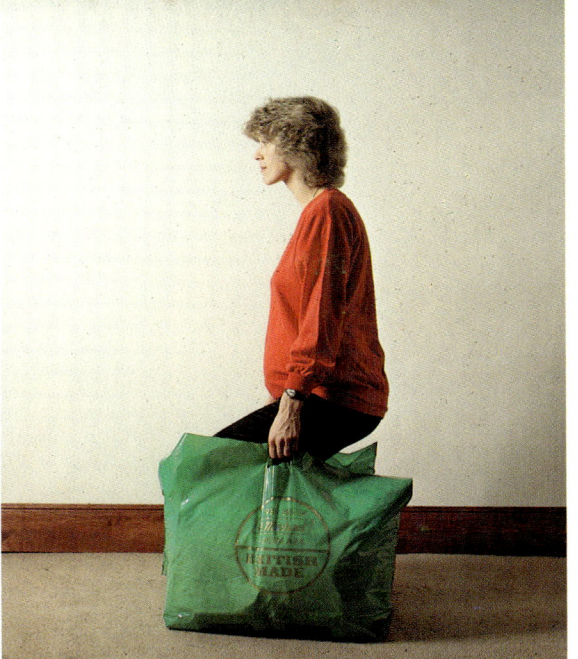

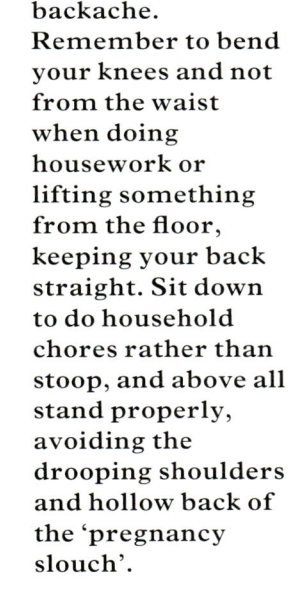

Good posture greatly reduces the strain on the spine that causes backache. Remember to bend your knees and not from the waist when doing housework or lifting something from the floor, keeping your back straight. Sit down to do household chores rather than stoop, and above all stand properly, avoiding the drooping shoulders and hollow back of the 'pregnancy slouch'.

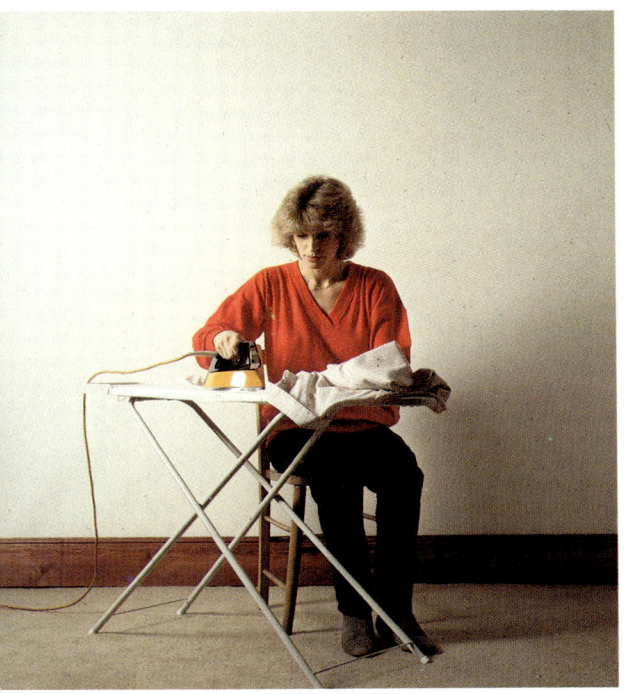

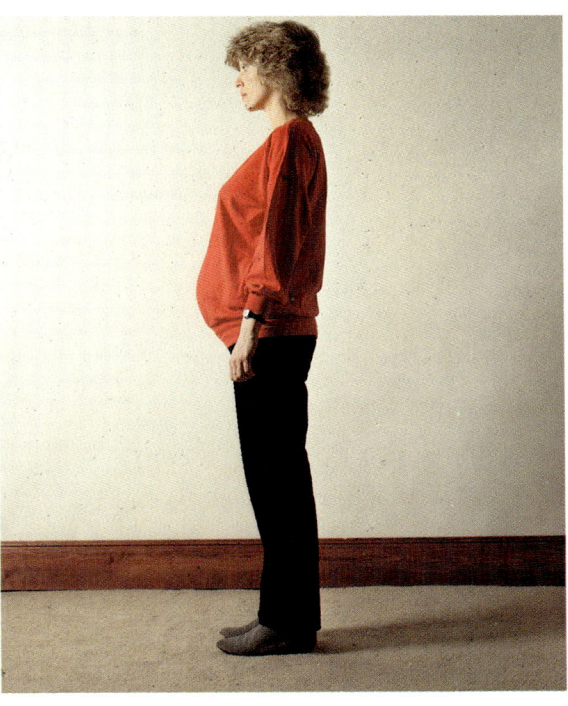

fades a few weeks after delivery.

If you are very fair-haired, you may suddenly notice a light down on your face – especially around the jaw-line – or abdomen, and even fairish hair on your arms and legs that you never thought you had. In fact this is not excess hair developing, it's just a darkening of the existing hair and will return to normal after the birth of your baby.

Occasionally a freckly, butterfly-shaped mask known as *chloasma* spreads over the face in late pregnancy and can be brought out if exposed to the sun or a solarium. If you sunbathe and notice a distinctive pattern – like a tea stain – forming from the nose, over your cheeks and on your forehead

it's as well to cover up straight away with a hat and keep your face completely shaded. The mask will fade with your tan but if established may never completely disappear.

However not all women get this type of pigmentation during pregnancy (darker women are again more prone), and one of the advantages of sunbathing – apart from the psychological boost of a suntan – is that the action of sunlight on the skin helps to form vitamin D in the body. But if you do sunbathe don't allow yourself to become too hot. Because of the increase in metabolic activity pregnant women tend to feel the heat more than usual and can be more susceptible to sunstroke, which is unpleasant under any circumstances.

Feet and ankles

During pregnancy a great strain is placed on the feet, again due to the softening and stretching of ligaments combined with your weight increase, and it's important to pay extra attention to them. Sit with your feet up whenever you can and never stand still for too long – this will cause your ankles and feet to swell as the blood gets down to them easily but has a lot of trouble getting back. The exercises below will help to keep the blood flowing freely. Ease aching feet by soaking them for ten to fifteen minutes in a bowl of salted tepid water.

Foot Massage

1 Sit comfortably on a chair with your back straight. Place the balls of your feet on a rolling pin, press them down and roll the pin backwards and forward – on a carpet is best.

2 Next tie your big toes together with a piece of tape (not too tight) then try to pull the feet apart. These are good exercises to do while watching television!

3 Still sitting – or else lying on the floor or in bed – rotate each foot in a circular motion, first to the left, then to the right. Take hold of each toe separately and wiggle it up and down as far as possible and then in a circular direction. These exercises help to loosen the joints as well as improving the circulation in the legs.

In some areas, chiropody is free for pregnant women and it's a good idea to take advantage of this perk if you can. A visit to a chiropodist every two months is a good idea, and more often than this towards the end of pregnancy. When manicuring your feet yourself, always cut the nails straight across and then round off the edges with a nail file. Your nails grow faster during pregnancy than at any other time, and if you cut down the sides or leave jagged corners you may find you have ingrowing toenails before too long. Massage dry and scaly skin regularly with an unperfumed hand or body lotion and use a pumice stone to rub off hard skin on the soles. Your feet will probably sweat more towards the end of pregnancy; if they do and the skin seems to be getting slightly soggy, make a habit of wiping in between the toes with a little surgical spirit to prevent this. Dusting with talc is *not* a good idea as it will just clog up the pores and make you sweat more than ever.

Varicose veins

Varicose veins can develop at any stage during pregnancy and are caused by the pressure of the enlarging uterus on the veins in the pelvis constricting the upward flow of blood from the legs to the heart. The veins in the legs may dilate and stretch if the

Feet need special attention during pregnancy. The foot massage exercises shown here take only a few minutes to do and will help prevent tired feet.

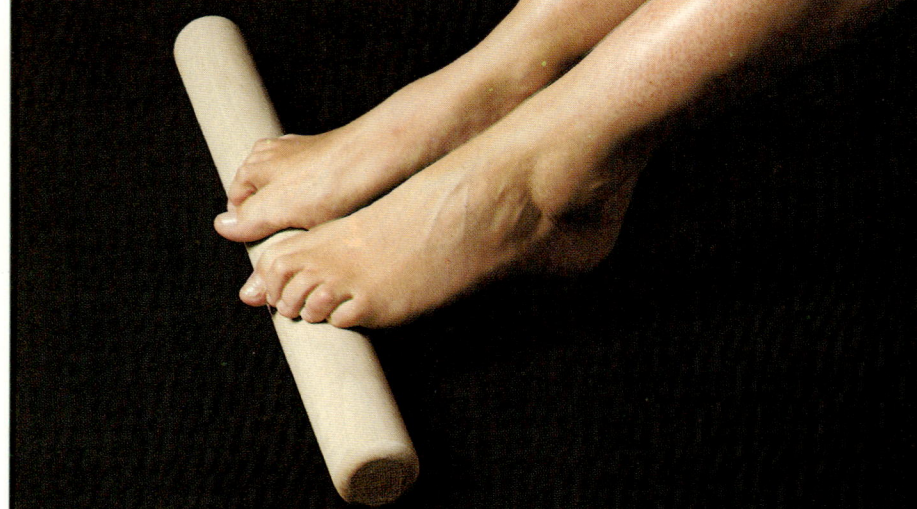

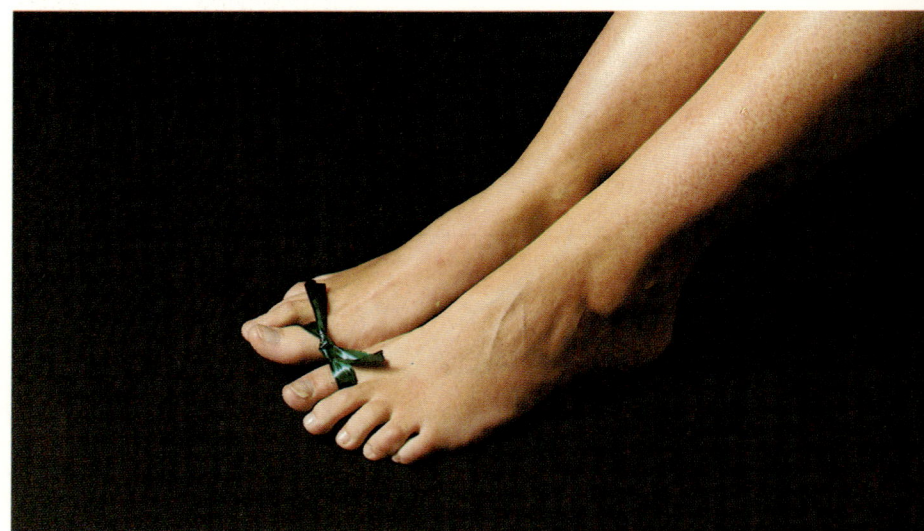

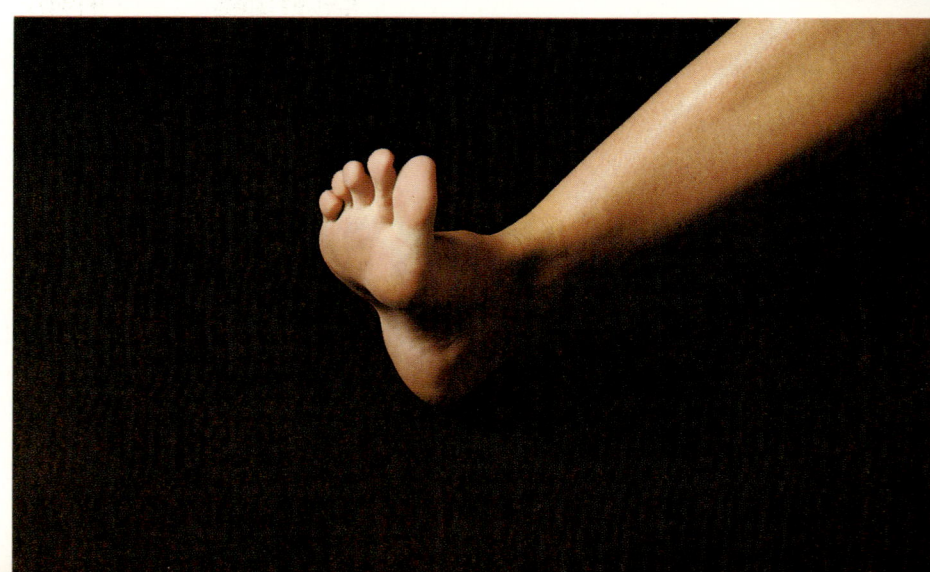

strain becomes too great and become painfully hard with a blue, lumpy appearance. There are usually warning signs before the veins appear: aching legs, cramp in the calves at night, swelling in the lower leg and around the ankle. Long hours of standing or sitting still (especially with the legs crossed), wearing elastic-topped socks or stockings or boots that are too tight, being overweight, and hereditary factors, can all contribute towards getting them.

Support tights worn from an early stage are the best way to ease or help to prevent varicose veins, but make sure they are not so tight that they cramp your feet. In some cases your doctor may prescribe support hose, but the medical varieties are usually rather drab and thick and guaranteed to make you feel dowdy. You can buy lightweight tights in flattering colours – the best of these contain a fibre called *Elastane* – which will look every bit as attractive as your normal tights or stockings. Put them on first thing in the morning, preferably even before you get out of bed or immediately after a bath, and wear them all day.

Varicose veins usually disappear after pregnancy when the weight is removed from the legs, but once you have suffered from them they will inevitably return with subsequent pregnancies. Try to avoid the problem by always sitting with your legs straight and uncrossed, if you cannot put them up. Don't sit for a long time in the same position – move your feet up or down – or stand in the same stance. Walk whenever possible – this will help maintain a steady flow of blood around the body. Also, watch your weight. The less bulk your legs have to carry, the less strain on the veins.

Vaginal discharges

There is an increase in mucus discharged from the vagina throughout pregnancy which, although you may find it annoying, is perfectly normal. However, if it begins to make you itch or causes an offensive smell, tell your doctor. You have probably developed a common fungus infection called thrush, which he will be able to deal with promptly. Hygiene is important, so take as many baths as you like – it is very rare for water to actually enter the vagina and even if it did it would certainly not infect it. Keep the area surrounding the vagina scrupulously clean during pregnancy, but always make sure you rinse away the soap. Wear cotton underwear, and when washing it take care that everything is well rinsed and no traces of soap powder have been left to cause irritation.

Teeth

It is very important to keep your teeth particularly clean during pregnancy. Extra hormones in the circulation make the gums much softer and unless you meticulously remove all the debris from between the teeth, the gums easily become damaged and then infected. This inflammation of the gums is called gingivitis. Gingivitis is common among non-pregnant people too but your gums are far more susceptible to infection at this time. If you notice that they bleed when you clean your teeth, it's likely that you have developed gingivitis. If you don't visit your dentist and have this remedied by thorough cleansing, your teeth will be more prone to decay than ever.

Cleanliness is the most important thing. Follow a strict regime of cleaning and dental flossing and visit your dentist for regular check-ups. Brush your teeth after every meal if possible with a medium or soft brush. Use dental floss daily to help remove food particles from between the teeth. If your gums do bleed, don't stop brushing them. Gentle friction will stimulate the gums and help release any trapped particles. Use a mouthwash to rinse these away.

Nails

Although their growth rate is invariably speeded up during pregnancy, nails may tend to become dry and brittle and split easily. Rub olive or baby oil into the base of the nails at night and massage – this should help to stimulate a stronger growth.

Eyes

Wearers of contact lenses may find that these become uncomfortable during pregnancy. This is because the shape of your eyeballs may change very slightly as a result of fluid retention. If they do then it is probably best to revert to wearing glasses until the eyes return to normal.

There is no reason why your eyesight should change during pregnancy. But if you do seem to be growing a little more short- or long-sighted than usual, don't change your lenses until after your baby is born.

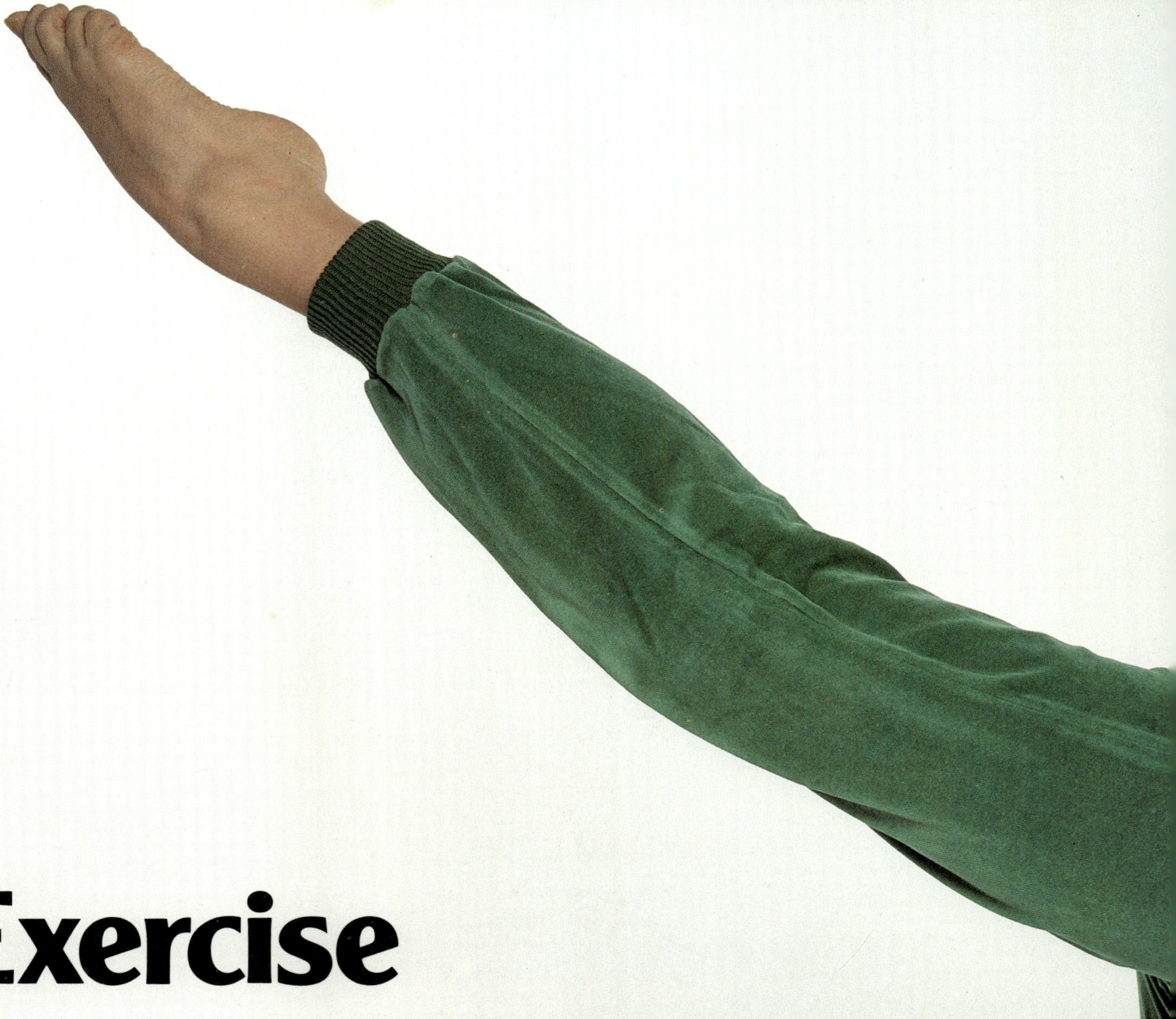

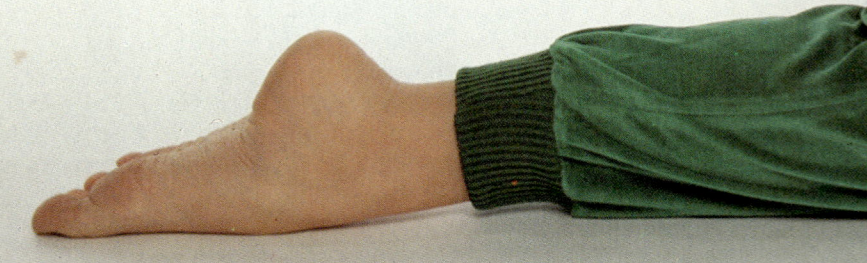

Exercise

Pregnancy is not an illness or a handicap, so there is no need to wrap yourself in cotton wool. On the whole, a sensible rule is to follow your habits rather than change them, but it's a pretty sure bet that if you make some attempt to keep your body exercised you'll feel much better for it – less lumpy and awkward – and find it easier to get back in trim after you have had the baby.

The kind of exercise you can do while pregnant depends very much on the sort of physical activity you have been used to before. If you have not previously played active games of tennis or squash, or attended keep-fit classes, this is hardly the time to start. The work of the heart may increase by as much as forty per cent by the twenty-eighth week. In fact, the heart itself enlarges with the increased load so don't give it extra, unnecessary work to do. Rest comes before exercise during pregnancy. If you have a home and other children to look after, you will automatically be kept fairly active. Washing floors, vacuuming and making beds are all vigorous duties and you should be careful not to over-tire yourself just with everyday housework.

However, if you are used to participating regularly in sports, there is no reason why you shouldn't continue throughout the first half of pregnancy – providing everything is progressing normally and your doctor agrees. There are obvious exceptions: water-skiing, snow-skiing, skin-diving and

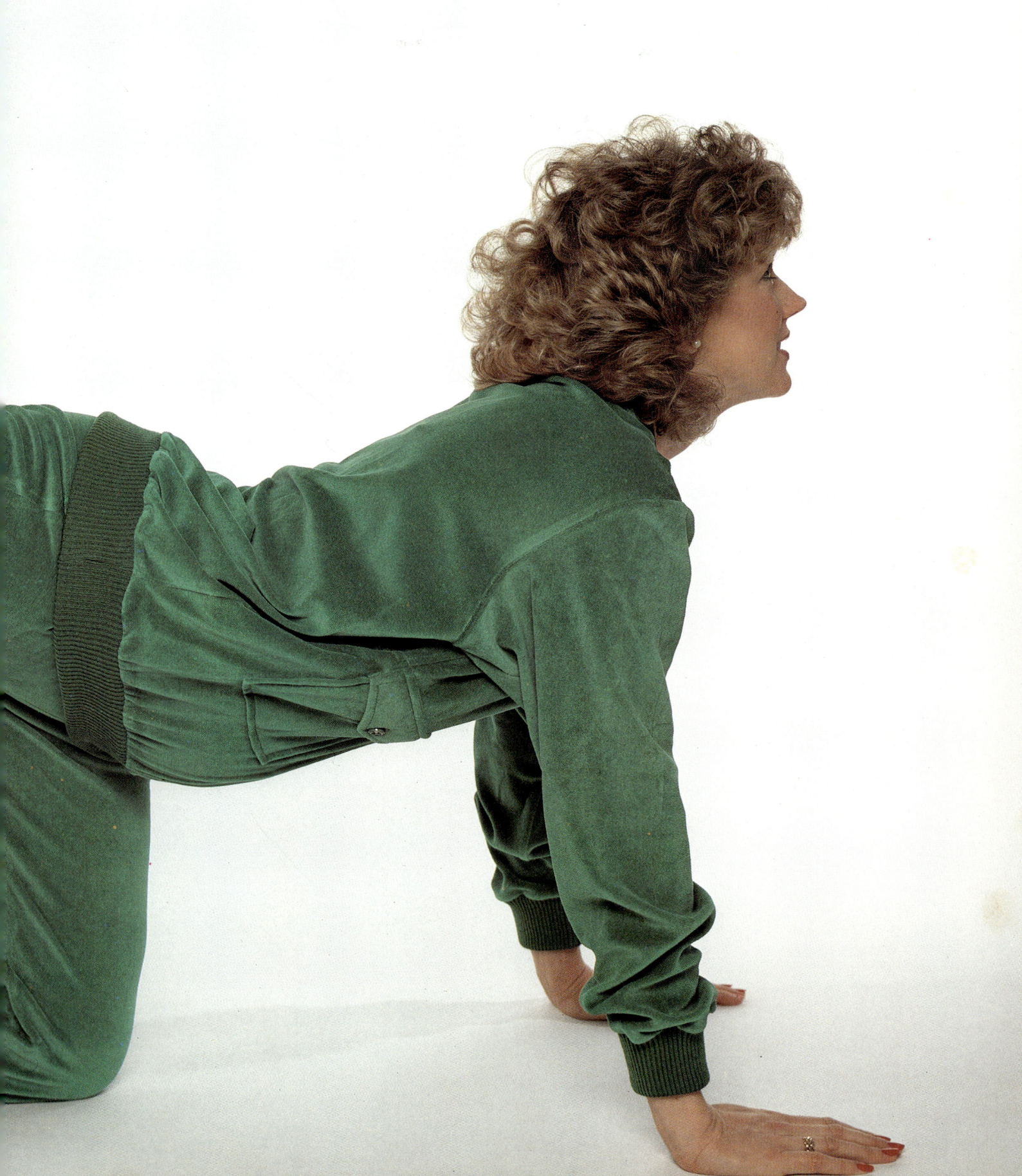

horse-riding are out since there is always a risk of injury. Cycling is fine as long as you are extremely careful not to tire yourself or to lose balance. In early pregnancy an accident could result in miscarriage and during the last few months the sheer bulk of the abdomen makes balancing precarious. By this stage it is very unlikely that any blow to the abdomen would actually harm the baby, but there is always a chance that the shock might bring on miscarriage or early labour. There is absolutely no excuse for not walking. Obviously mountaineering, cross-country runs and hiking are not advisable, but walking short distances – getting to and from work, for example – rather than taking the bus or driving, can only help you keep fit so long as you don't exhaust yourself. The same is true of dancing – it's good for you providing it's not too acrobatic. The amount of energy involved in your dancing will depend entirely on how you feel, and of course, your weight will dictate how late into your pregnancy you wish to continue. It is unlikely that you will feel much like leaping around in a discothèque during the last two or three months.

Swimming is fine – so long as you don't allow yourself to become out of breath and over-tired. But if you are not used to swimming you should avoid it during the first three months. Never swim in very cold water as you are more likely to get cramp, and don't try any high diving. Only experienced divers should even attempt to dive and then only from heights of three feet or less, as the sudden change in your blood pressure could affect the baby's circulation. Check with your doctor before embarking on an exercise programme – if you have a history of miscarriage he may not advise it. The exercises on the following pages are simple and medically approved, and will gently tone up your body during pregnancy whether you have exercised before or not. Don't be complacent and leave it all until after the birth – it might be too late then. Aim to go into labour with your body supple and trim.

Work out on a blanket or heavy towel if the floor is too hard, and wear loose-fitting garments – a leotard is all right if it stretches enough but don't wear one if it's constricting. All these exercises are safe to do throughout pregnancy, but stop at once if a position becomes uncomfortable or hurts, and take particular care in the first few weeks.

Exercise Programme

Relaxation

Begin your programme with these simple breathing exercises for relaxation, especially if you have never exercised before. Remember whenever you get up off the floor to roll on to your side first.

Hand press
Stand straight with your hands together in a prayer position in front of your chest, shoulders dropped and elbows lifted outwards. Breathe in (slightly slower than normal breathing), expanding your stomach. Then breathe out, pulling your stomach in and pressing the palms of your hands together as hard as possible. Repeat ten to twenty times. Apart from being relaxing, this exercise is good for your stomach muscles, breasts and upper arms.

Deep breathing
Lie on your back on the floor in a relaxed position with your knees bent upwards and feet slightly apart, and with your hands resting on your stomach. Breathe in slowly, making the breath as long as you can manage, and expanding the stomach – feel it rise with your fingers. Then breathe out slowly, emptying your lungs, pulling your stomach flat, and pressing the small of your back into the floor. Start by breathing out to a count of five and work up to ten. Repeat

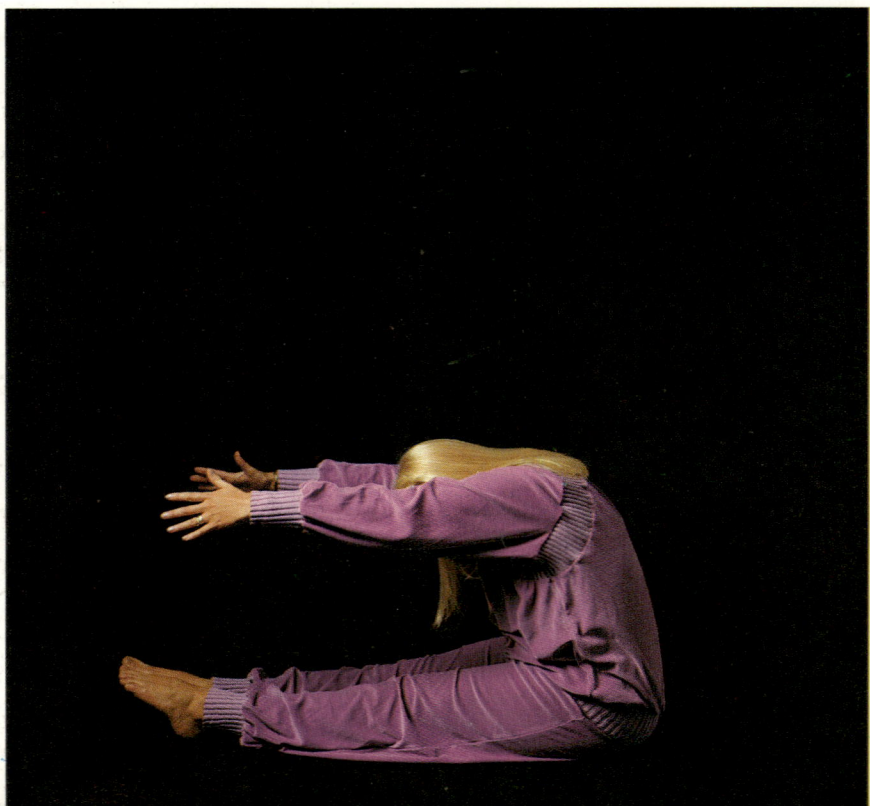

the exercise ten to twenty times. It is also good for your tummy.

Stretch
Sit on the floor with your legs stretched out in front of you, knees together and back straight but relaxed. Breathe in, lowering your chin forward so that you lengthen your spine, but keep it straight, at the same time reaching upwards with your arms – the palms facing each other and fingers splayed. Keeping your legs straight (knees pressed into the ground) and arms in the same position, stretch out forward from the base of the spine, simultaneously breathing out and pulling in your stomach. Lean as far as you can over your legs and hold it for a few seconds before returning to the upright position. Repeat ten to twenty times. This is both a relaxing and stretching exercise; you won't of course be able to reach so far forward during the later stages of pregnancy.

Back stretch
Lie on your back with your knees bent up so that your feet are flat on the floor and slightly apart, and your arms stretched back above your head. Keeping your arms relaxed, breathe in, expanding your stomach and arching your back slightly off the floor. Then breathe out all your air, pulling the back of your waist into the floor so that your tailbone lifts very slightly, and stretching your arms out backwards as far as you can. Repeat ten to twenty times. This stretch complements the previous exercise.

Toning up

The following tone-up exercises are for the pelvis, abdomen, back, legs, arms, bottom and breasts.

Pelvic tilt
To tone up the muscles of the pelvic area and abdomen, lie flat on the floor with your legs bent, knees together, feet slightly apart, and arms by your sides. Arch your back slightly. Then push the small of your back into the floor and tighten your buttock muscles. As you do this you will feel your tummy muscles gently tighten also. Relax back into the first position and repeat ten times. This exercise is particularly good for relieving backache.

Leg stretch
Using a chair, mantelpiece or doorknob for support, stand sideways to this with your back and legs straight, feet together. Balance your weight on the leg nearest your support and lift the outside leg a few inches from the ground in front of you – or higher if you can – keeping the toes pointed. Bend and straighten the knee six times. Then turn round and repeat with the other leg.

Bottom toner
Lie on the floor with your legs bent, feet apart, and arms by your sides. Raise your bottom slightly off the floor so that the weight of your body is supported by the upper part of your back. Tighten and relax

Far left: Stretch, a relaxation exercise. Centre and below: Leg stretch and Bottom toner, two exercises for toning you up.

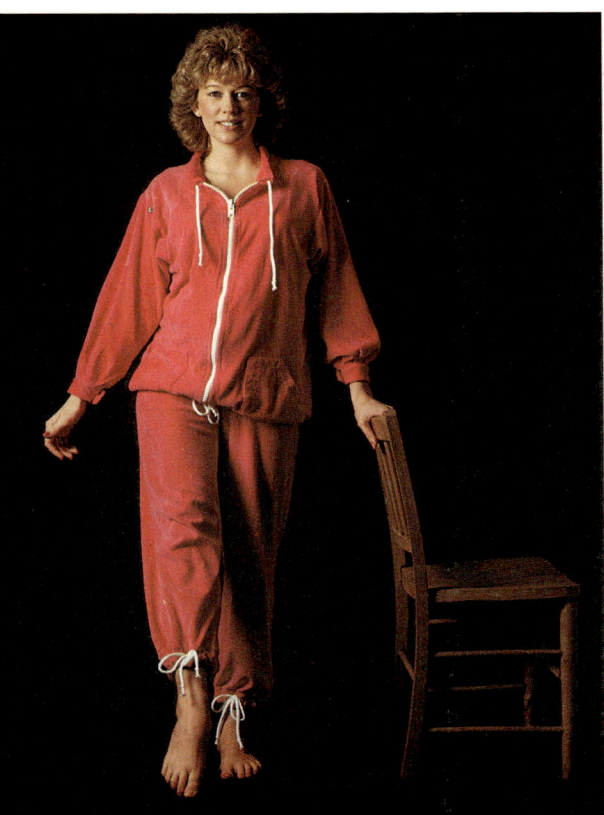

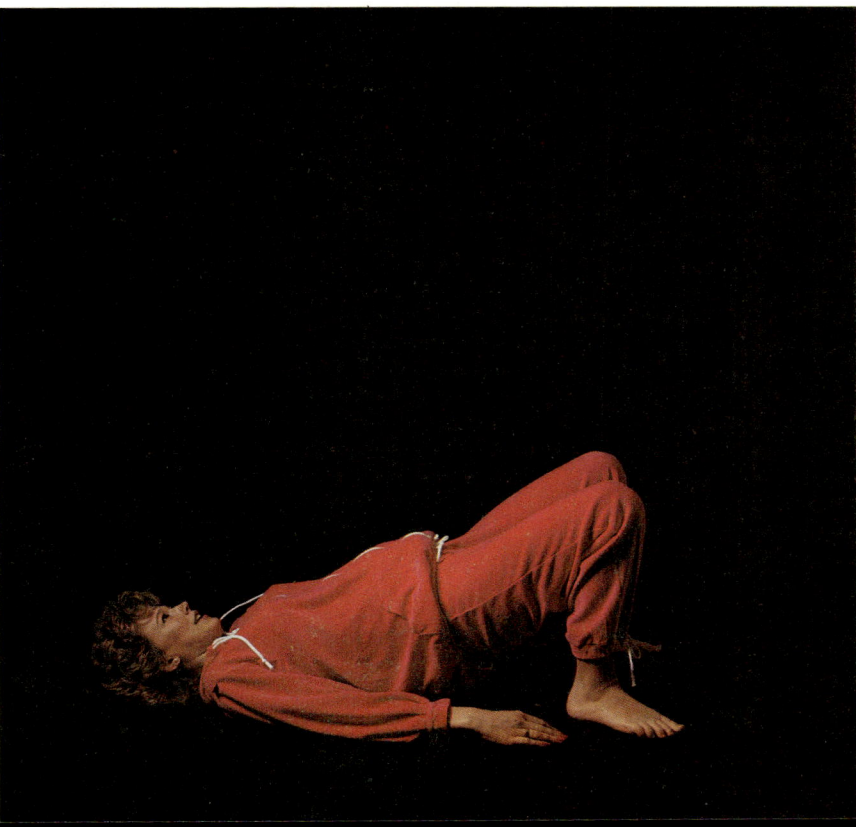

the buttock muscles, thirty times to start with, but try to work up to a hundred if you can. This is only a little movement, the hips should not move much, but it is an excellent exercise for toning the pelvic area and stomach.

Breasts
Stand straight and hold your left wrist with the right hand and your right wrist with the left hand, palms facing. Keep your wrists away from your body and raise your arms to chin level – the higher the better. Holding firmly, push the hands towards your elbows in short, sharp movements – thirty times or as many as you can comfortably manage. Move your arms up and down as you do this exercise, from chin to eye level.

Upper arms
Still standing, hold your arms straight out to the sides at right angles to your body. Clench your fists to tense the arms. Then rotate both arms together in small, tight circles backwards twenty times, then twenty times forwards.

Scissors in the air
Lie flat on your back and bend your knees up towards your chin. Hold on to your thighs and curl the top part of your body forward towards your knees so that your head and shoulders come off the floor.

Straighten your legs out completely; let go of your thighs and stretch your arms to the ceiling. You should now be stretching upwards with legs, arms and head.

Keeping your legs very straight (toes either pointed or flexed towards you) make large, slow strides up and down in the air without quite touching the ground. This is a smooth, sweeping scissor action, don't jerk. Start with ten and see if you can build up to fifty scissors. This exercise is very good for the stomach and legs.

Back arch
Kneel on all fours with your arms straight and directly under your shoulders. Breathe out all your air, humping up your back, pulling your stomach into your backbone, and letting your head drop right forward – try to touch your chest with your chin. Then breathe in deeply, pushing your bottom into the air, arching your back and lifting your head up and back so that you can look at the ceiling. Repeat this whole movement up to six times. This exercise is for the spine, stomach and pelvic area, and is another good one for relieving backache.

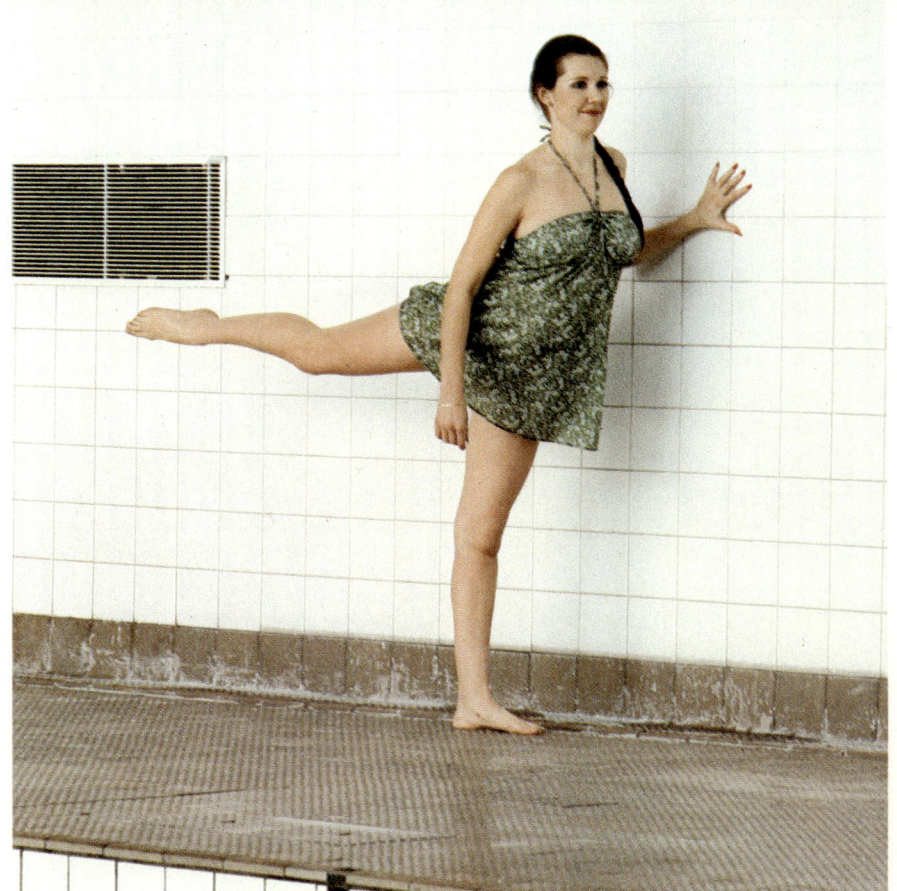

Swimming pool exercises

Even though you may not be keen on swimming or cannot swim at all, going to your local baths can provide one of the best ways to tone up your body and give it exercise during pregnancy – as well as making you feel good. As you become heavier you will find it a blessing to float in the water. The bulk that makes you feel as though you are carrying a sack of potatoes won't burden you at all because the water takes your weight. Another bonus is that if you have children, visiting your local baths makes a pleasurable outing for them too. A note of caution – taking to the water, as with all forms of exercise, should never be attempted after a heavy meal.

Leg warm-ups
Stand in the pool at a depth where the water is just below your bust. Fold your arms under the breasts to support them and run on the spot. Let the pressure of the water gently massage your legs and get the circulation going. Do thirty runs – or as many as you like.

Arm warm-ups
Stand in the pool with just your head and shoulders above the water. Keeping your

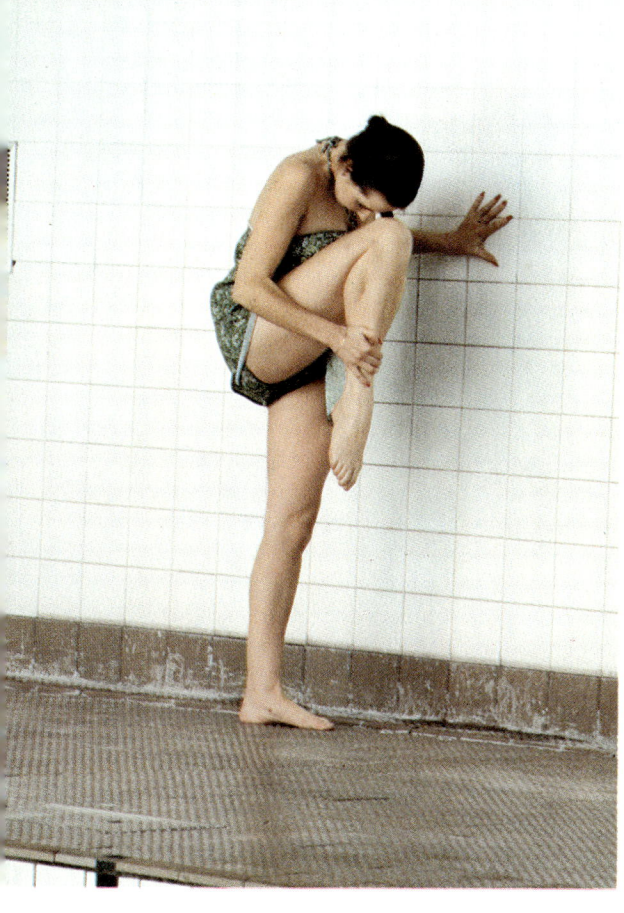

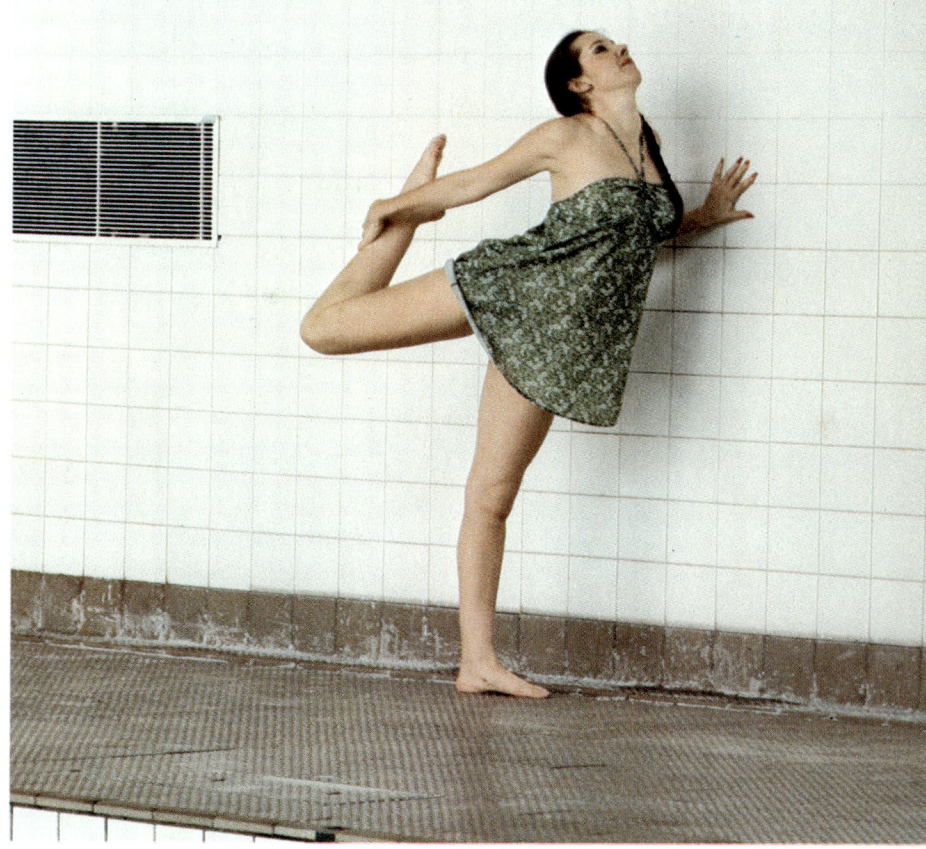

arms under and straight out in front of you, lean forward and pummel the water with clenched fists, as though it were a punch bag. This will help the circulation and tone the upper arms. Do at least thirty pummels, or more if you want to.

Water windmills
A good exercise for the shoulder joints is to stand in the pool with the shoulders just under water. Keeping the arms straight, rotate the left arm backwards in a full circle six times, as if you were doing backstroke. Repeat with the right arm, then change direction and rotate each arm forwards six times.

Leg swings
Stand at the side of the pool, sideways on and holding on to the wall with one hand, the water at bust level. Keeping both legs straight, swing the outside leg forward and back six times, getting the leg as high as possible. Turn round and swing the other leg forward and back six times. Repeat with each leg.

Leg rotations
Standing in the same position holding on to the side of the pool, raise the outside leg and, keeping it straight, rotate it in a large circle – front, side, back. Do this six times,

then reverse the circle – back, side, front, for another six rotations. Turn round and repeat with the other leg.

Water cycling
Stand with your back against the side of the pool, stretching out your arms to hold on to the side. Let your body float out in front of you and 'bicycle' with your legs for as long as you want.

Spine stretch
Stand sideways to the wall holding on with one hand, water at about waist level. Bend your outside knee and clasp hold of the ankle. Then push the knee forwards and up in front of you, leaning the head and shoulders forward in an effort to meet it. Now pull the bent leg behind you and, leaning the top half of your body backwards with the head thrown back, very gently stretch the spine. Do this exercise six times, then turn round and repeat with the other leg.

Walking up the wall
Turn round to face the wall and hold the bar or ledge with both hands. Keeping the legs straight, walk up the side of the pool to meet your hands, then walk down again. Repeat this several times; it is a good stretching exercise for the spine and the backs of the thighs.

Swimming pool exercises can be rather more athletic because the water will support your weight: Leg swings (far left), Spine stretch (centre and above).

Yoga

As with all exercises, you should check with your doctor before taking up yoga when you are pregnant, however simple the poses look. These positions are specially designed for pregnant women and, unless you have a history of miscarriage, will be safe to do throughout pregnancy.

Mountain pose
Stand straight with your feet together. Don't lean over your toes, but keep your weight evenly distributed between the balls of your feet and your heels. Stretch your whole body up towards the ceiling as though the top of your head was attached to it by a string. Keep your chin down slightly and let your shoulders relax, holding them back and down at the same time. Breathe deeply.

Baddha Konasana
Sit on the floor with your back against a wall, and bring the soles and heels of your feet together. Catch hold of your toes with your hands, straighten your back, then press your knees downwards towards the floor so that your thighs open wider. Hold your legs in this position for as long as you can – try to work the time up from say ten seconds to a few minutes.

Virasana (Hero pose)
Kneel down with your feet on either side of your buttocks, which should be resting on the floor (if necessary support them with a cushion). Make sure your toes are pointing backwards as far as you can so that you feel the stretch along your legs, and keep your back straight. Lift your hands above your head, intertwining your fingers, and hold for a few minutes. This is a lovely open upward stretch that really feels good as well as being excellent for toning the spine and pelvic area and also relaxing for tired legs.

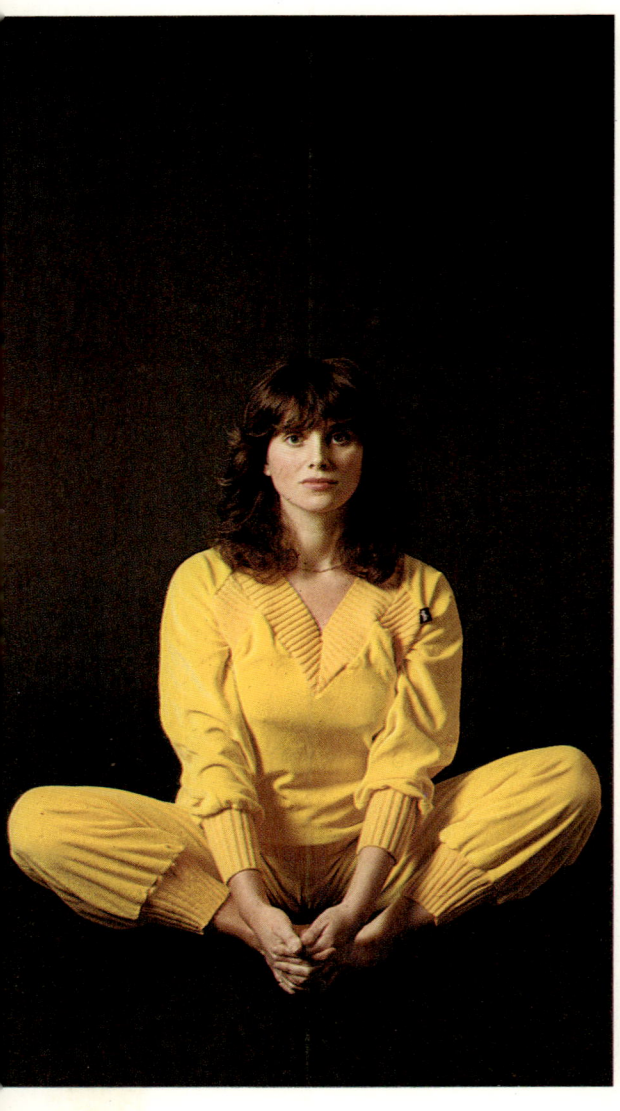

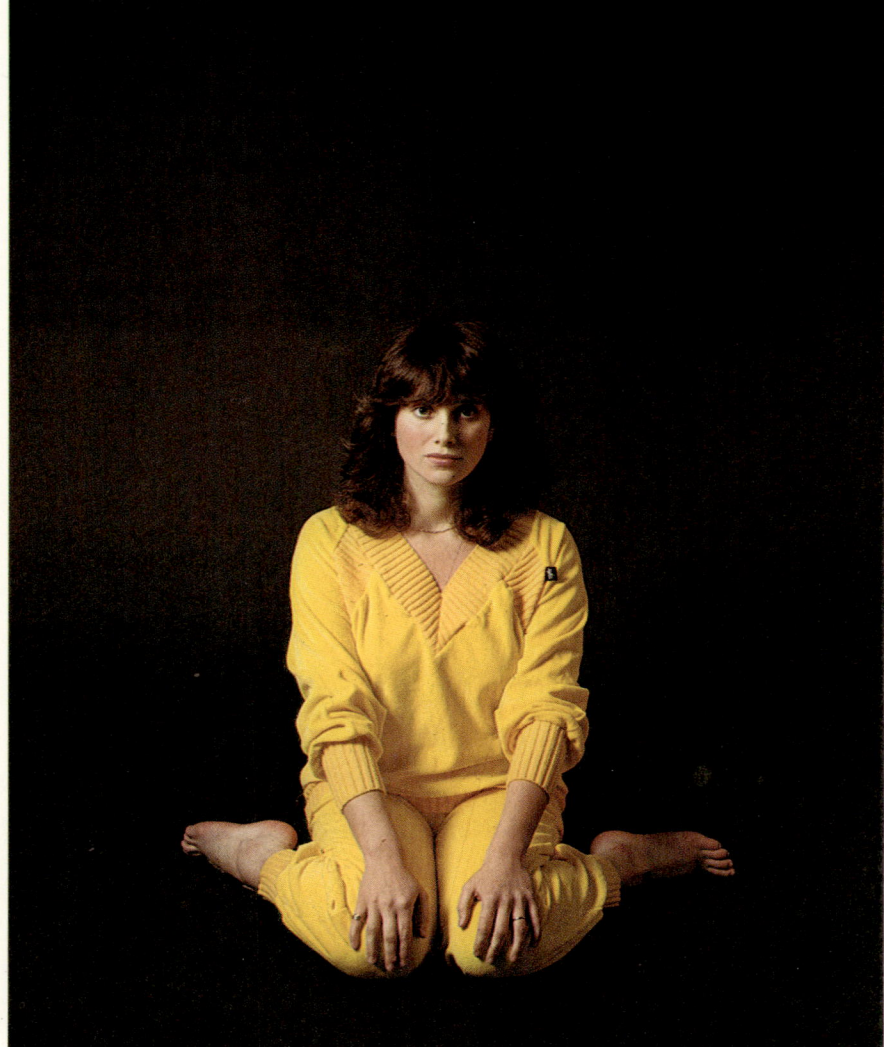

Squatting

Stand with your feet about eighteen inches to two feet apart, toes pointing slightly outward. Then crouch down in a squatting position keeping the feet flat (go on to your toes if you can't manage this at first), knees out and the back straight. Hold on to a support (the arms of a low chair, for instance) to begin with if you need to. Stay squatting for about a minute to start with, but try and work up to five minutes, and go into it when you can throughout the day. This 'birth' position helps to stretch the muscles of the pelvic floor in preparation for labour, it is most important to practise it right from the beginning of pregnancy until the very end.

Savasana (Corpse pose)

Lie on your back with your eyes closed (check you are lying in a straight line), legs slightly apart and your arms resting at about an angle of forty-five degrees to your body, and with the palms upwards. Your spine should be flat on the floor – if you find this uncomfortable or difficult, try placing a cushion under your thighs.

Now, starting with your feet, go through each part of your body slowly tensing and relaxing it (imagine your tensions and worries disappearing as you do so). Flex your toes up towards you, and relax them so they fall outward. Tighten and relax your calves, knees, thighs, buttocks and stomach – try and make it touch your backbone. Make fists with your hands and relax them, tighten and relax your arms, raise your shoulders and let them sink back, lift your head and let it relax back. Screw up your face and relax it, keeping your mouth slightly open so that the jaw is relaxed.

Having relaxed your body, now concentrate on nice, slow, rhythmical breathing. Breathe in, filling your lungs and expanding your stomach, and breathe out emptying them. Continue to lie in this position for as long as you like or have time for. It is a good way to end an exercise session and is also very useful if sleeping becomes difficult in the later months.

Three yoga positions suited for pregnant women are Baddha Konasana (far left), Virasana (centre two), and the Squatting position (below).

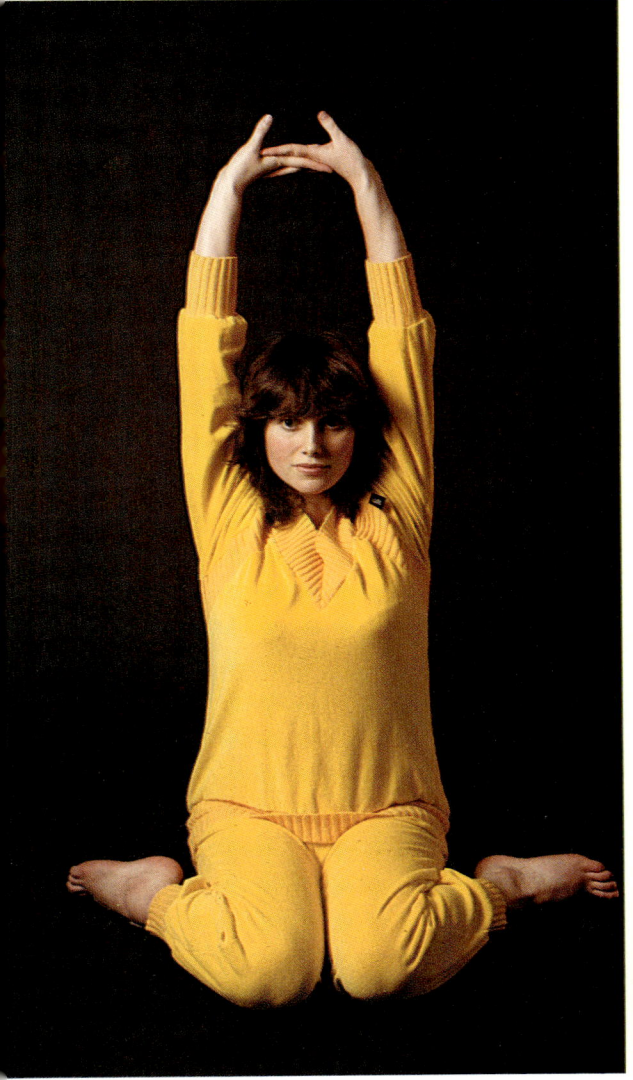

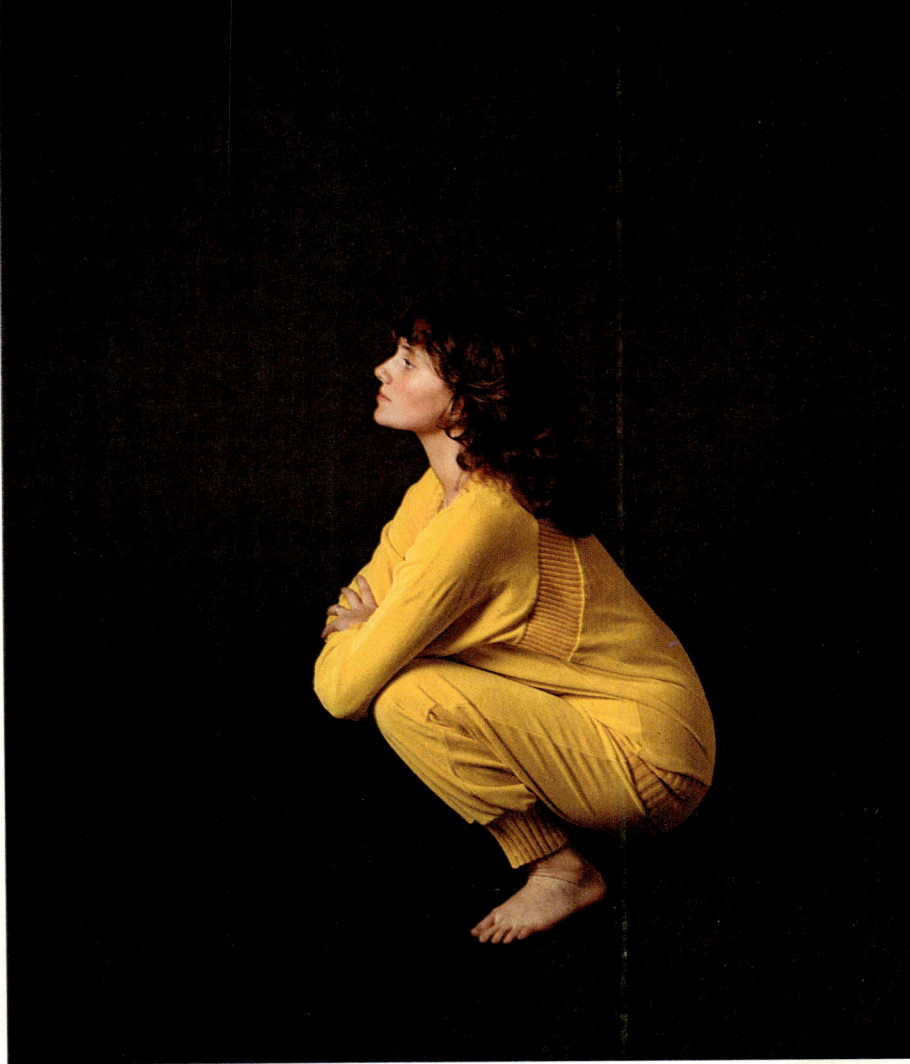

Diet and Weight

The old saying 'eating for two' is definitely out of date and anyone who suggests that this is what you should be doing can be politely ignored. It used to be thought that a fat, bouncing baby was a healthy baby. Now we know that fat children often become fat adults and that obesity can lead to heart disease. However, there will be a natural increase in your appetite during pregnancy, which you should not deny providing you don't satisfy it with too many refined and processed foods. A well-balanced diet is important throughout life, but particularly so during pregnancy when you have to satisfy your baby's nutritional requirements as well as your own. So make sure you are eating wisely and well.

It is not healthy for anyone to be overweight – or underweight – and the importance of keeping your weight under control cannot be over-stressed. A large weight gain during pregnancy may give rise to high blood pressure, swelling of the feet and ankles and undue strain on the heart. It can also be very hard to lose the excess fat after the birth.

Most doctors these days watch weight gain keenly. Every time you attend the antenatal clinic you will be weighed and if the doctor feels you are putting on too much he will advise you to cut down on starchy foods. If he is worried about the amount of weight you have put on, he will almost certainly recommend a strict diet plan which it is sensible to follow.

On average, a woman on a well-balanced diet will put on around 11–12.5 kg (24–28 lb) during her pregnancy (although some women may put on a lot more or less than this). The gain is due to the combined weight of the baby, placenta, increasing blood supply to the uterus (which at full term is about twenty-five per cent of the total body circulation), amniotic fluid

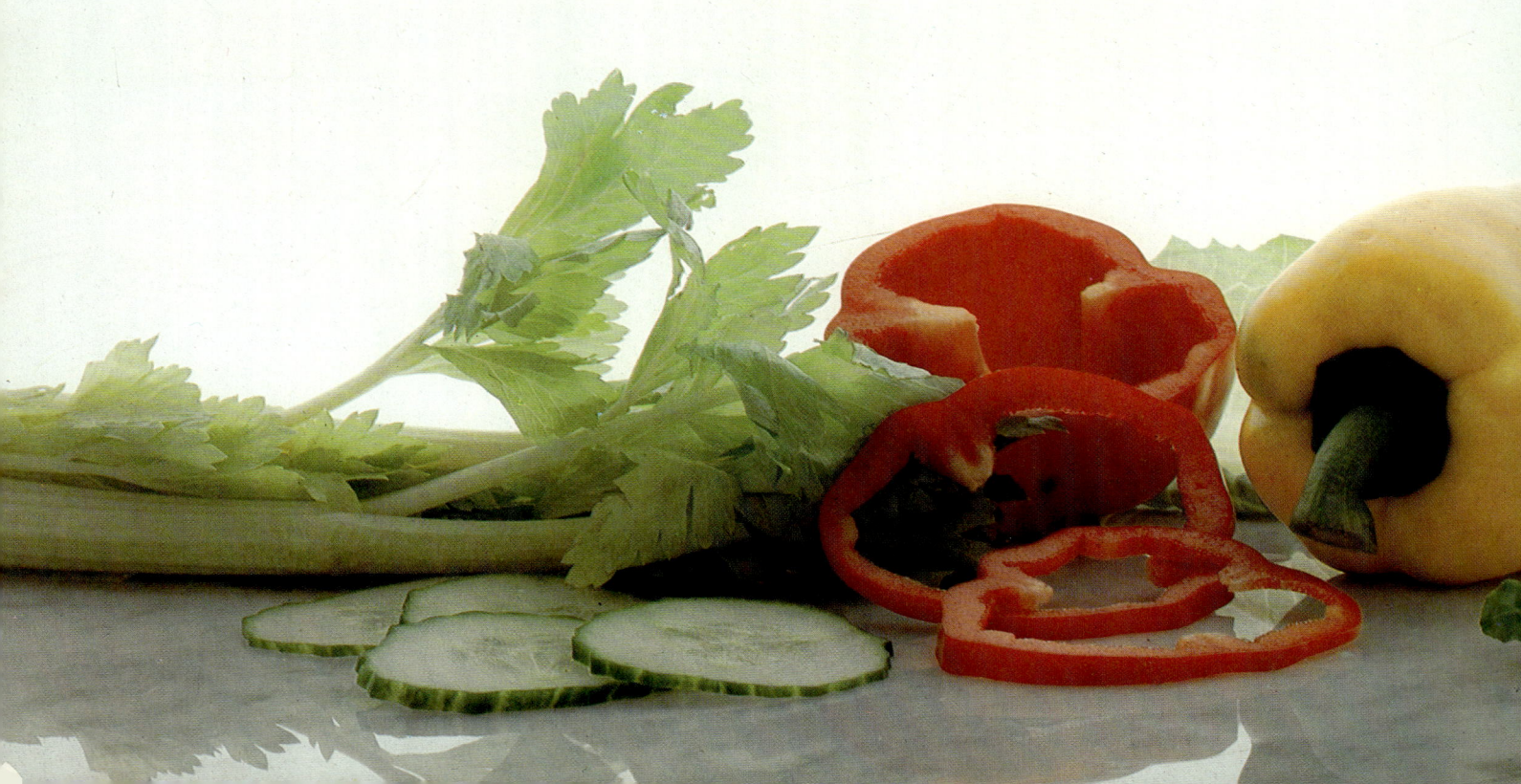

around the baby, water retention, plus a natural increase in fat reserves and the enlargement of various organs such as the breasts and the uterus. Although some pregnancy guide books advise a lesser weight gain in the region of 8–9 kg (18–20 lb) most doctors feel that about 12.5 kg (28 lb) shows a healthy, normal average.

There are plenty of misunderstandings

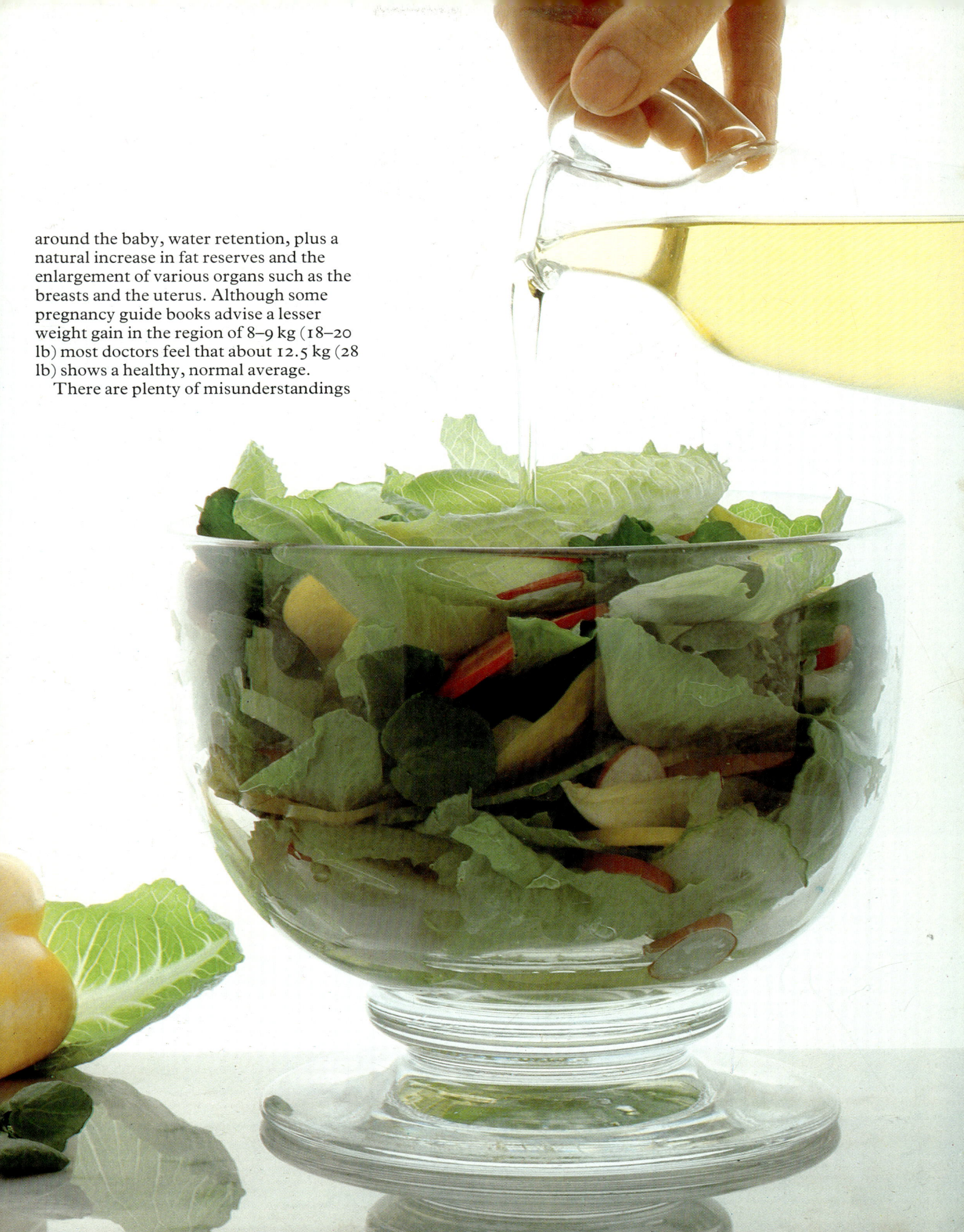

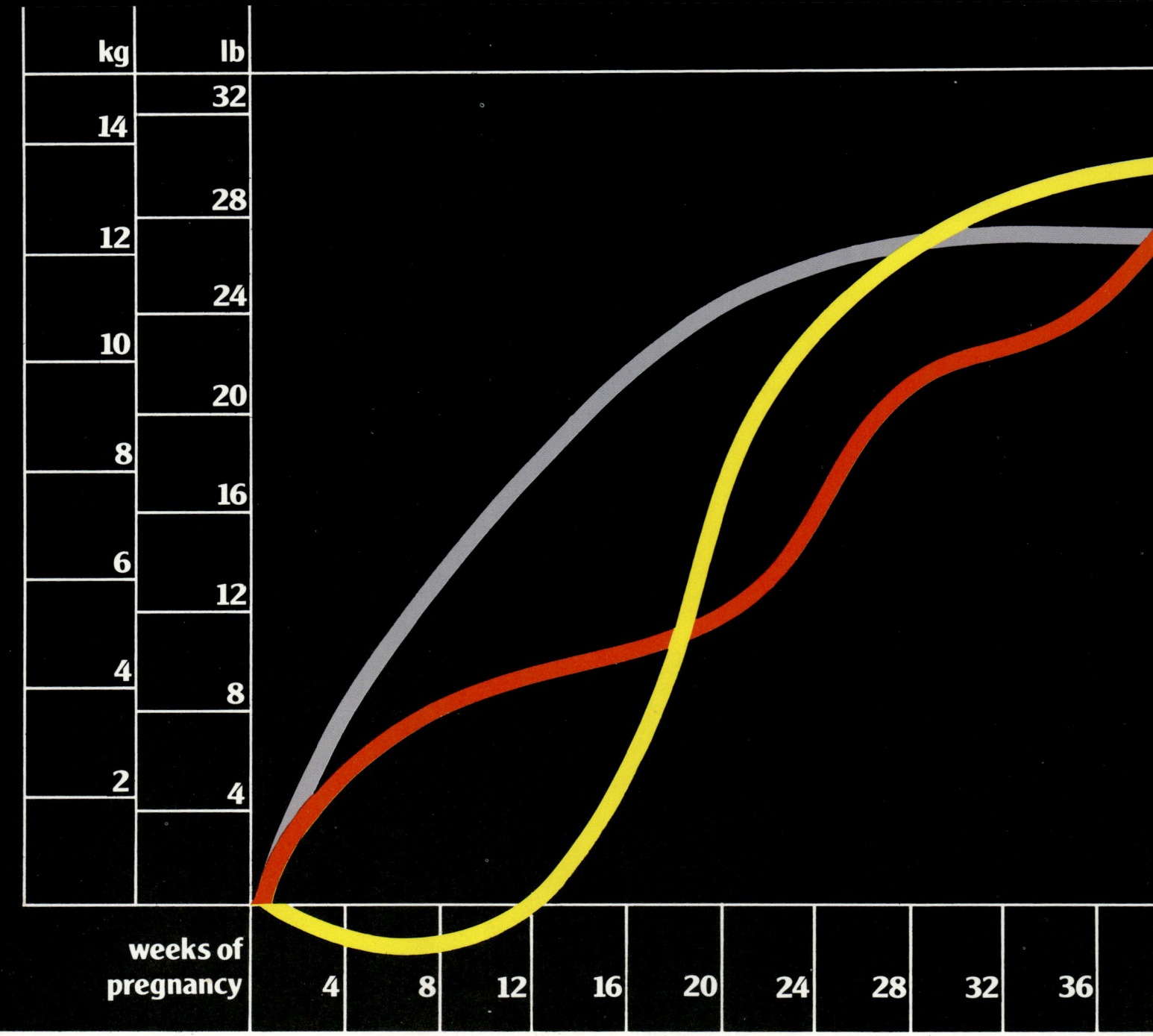

kg	lb									
	32									
14										
	28									
12										
	24									
10										
	20									
8										
	16									
6										
	12									
4										
	8									
2										
	4									
weeks of pregnancy		4	8	12	16	20	24	28	32	36

about the pattern of weight gain during pregnancy and for weight-conscious women this can be a source of worry. You will notice a difference in your general shape apart from the obvious 'tummy'. The face tends to get fuller especially around the cheeks, jowls and neck, the shoulders thicken, as does the waistline. A little extra padding may be noticeable around the lower back, thighs and bottom. This increase in stored fat is quite normal and is laid down as an energy deposit in preparation for breastfeeding. It is easy to feel despondent as your clothes get tighter and tighter in places you hadn't expected, but don't fight this natural weight increase. Going on crash or fad diets while pregnant can certainly be harmful to both you and the baby. What

you must remember is, everyone is different and whereas some people don't start putting on weight until about fourteen weeks or so, others find the scales shoot up immediately. Often it is the thinner women who put on most weight and fairly early on, whereas women who are overweight to start with gain comparatively little throughout their pregnancy.

You may like to check your own weight every week to chart your gain. But if you do seem to be putting on too much too soon – it should average between quarter and half a kilo ($\frac{1}{2}$–1 lb) a week – don't panic. Think about your diet. Are you eating too much refined food? If so, cut out fattening cakes and if you feel hungry between meals, nibble fruit and raw vegetables such as

Patterns of weight gain can vary enormously, even for healthy normal pregnancies. So while many women put on weight more or less steadily throughout the nine months (red line), some may actually lose a few pounds initially (yellow line) due to morning sickness, catching up again later, while others may begin well, but then lose weight towards the end of term when the baby puts on a sudden spurt of growth and uses up the mothers reserves (blue line).

carrots or celery. A plain biscuit or slice of lightly buttered toast won't make much difference but frequent chocolate bars or jam doughnuts will.

Sensible planning of your meals throughout the day will ensure that you and your baby get all the vitamins, minerals and nutrients needed. On the next page is a list of the essential nutrients that make up a well-balanced diet and, most important, help ensure a healthy baby.

How to keep a balanced diet

The important thing in maintaining a well-balanced diet is not to eat too much of any one type of food: you need variety in order to get adequate supplies of essential protein, minerals and vitamins. Try to keep the same kind of balance of these in your diet as before you were pregnant – about 2,500 calories daily should be sufficient for your energy needs. If you eat too many refined carbohydrates, found for example in cakes, sweets, and soft drinks, your calorie intake will become excessive and the body's metabolism simply won't be able to burn up the calories fast enough.

You can make sure of getting all the necessary nutrients by planning your daily meals from the following four basic groups. Try to eat as many fresh and untreated foods as possible, as the processing and heat treatments used to produce 'convenience' foods considerably reduce their nutritional value.

Dairy products
Milk is the best dairy product, as it is high in protein and calcium, and you should try to have a pint a day. Skimmed milk is less nutritious as it has lost essential fatty acids, which are important as vitamins. So if you are worried about your weight half a pint of whole milk is still better for you than to substitute skimmed milk. Cheese is fairly rich in protein and calcium and contains vitamins A and D, but is also high in fat. Cottage cheese is a nutritious alternative. Butter and margarine are another source of vitamins A and D. If you have a small appetite or don't like drinking milk, a good quality dairy ice cream is rich in calcium, carbohydrate and fats, so a small portion would make an ideal dessert. Avoid the commercial varieties described as non-dairy produce, as they contain dubious fats rather than milk, plus chemicals and additives.

Cream is high in calcium and protein – and fat. For those who dislike milk, natural yoghurt makes a good nutritional substitute, as it is high in calcium.

Meat, fish and eggs
Offal (liver, kidneys and heart) is an excellent source of protein, iron and B vitamins. It is especially good for you if you are anaemic and essential if, for any reason, you are not taking iron tablets. Red meats (beef, lamb and pure beef hamburgers) also contain a lot of protein and iron. Poultry (chicken and turkey) has a high protein content, and roasting is a good way to cook the meat without losing the goodness. White fish (cod, haddock, halibut, sole etc.) are similar in nutritional value to poultry. Tinned fish (pilchards, sardines, tuna and herring) are rich in calcium, iron, vitamin A and protein, but they tend to be oily so their calorie content is higher. Eggs too, are a good source of protein, calcium, fat and vitamins A and D.

Bread and cereals
All bread contains calcium, carbohydrate, iron and protein. However processed bread contains 'empty calories' which means that you are getting more stodge and fewer nutrients than you will in wholemeal bread – which is also a good source of roughage. Whole cereals contain similar nutrients to wholemeal bread. Pasta and rice products contain carbohydrates, calcium and iron, and are not as fattening as is generally assumed – it's the rich sauces served with the pasta and the creamy milk in the rice puddings that do the calorific damage. Again brown rice and pasta are better for you than white.

Vegetables and fruit
Dried beans and peas are a cheap source of protein. Green vegetables and potatoes are high in vitamin C and a major source of dietary fibre. Vegetables are best eaten raw or steamed to avoid nutrient losses during cooking, and potatoes are most nourishing cooked and eaten in their jackets. Spinach, haricot beans and lentils are high in calcium and iron. Carrots are a valuable source of vitamin A. Blackcurrants, oranges, lemons and grapefruit are rich in vitamin C. Try to eat some of the pith of citrus fruits, too, as this is exceptionally high in vitamin content. 'Fleshy' fruits such as bananas and mangoes are less plentiful in vitamins but contain carbohydrate. Dried fruits such as currants, sultanas and dates contain concentrated sugar and are a valuable source of energy.

What you need

It is particularly important when you are pregnant to include in your diet adequate amounts of all the essential nutrients, vitamins and minerals. These are listed below together with their chief functions and main food sources.

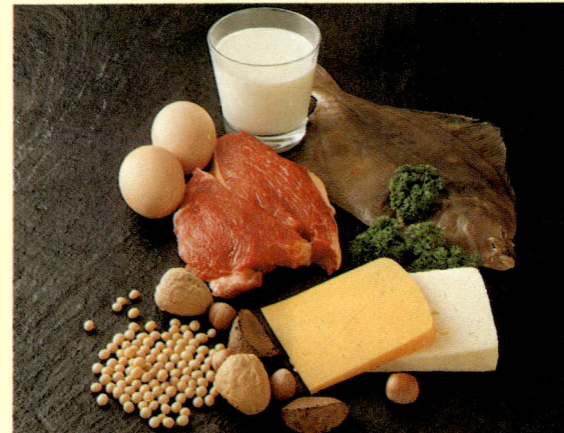

PROTEIN is tissue-building and therefore essential for your baby's growth, a healthy placenta and uterus. It also keeps your blood sugar level high which will help prevent depression. Main sources: meat, fish, eggs, milk, cheese, soya beans, nuts, pulses.

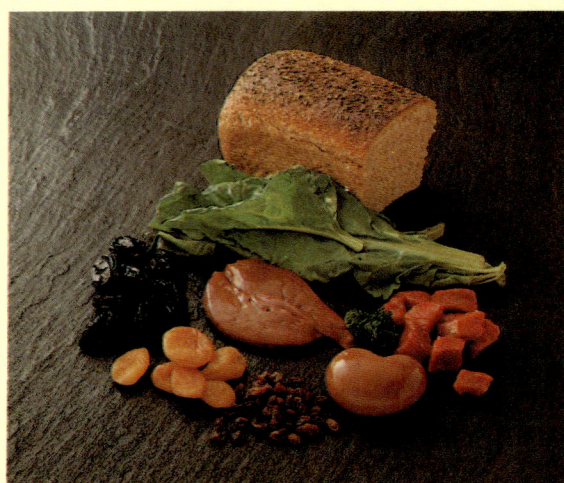

IRON increases the number of red cells in the blood and will stop you becoming anaemic as your blood increases in volume and therefore tends to thin. It will also stand you in good stead if you lose blood during delivery. Main sources: liver, beef, kidney, cocoa powder, green vegetables, watercress, dried fruit, wholemeal bread. Your doctor will probably also prescribe iron tablets.

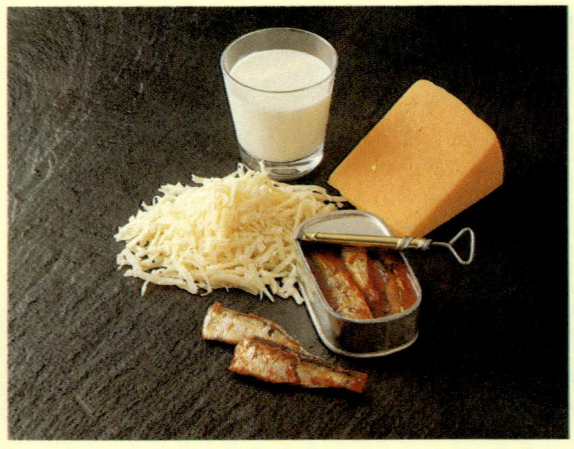

CALCIUM is important for the development of your baby's teeth and bones. Main sources: milk, cheese, bones of tinned little fish, i.e. sardines, pilchards.

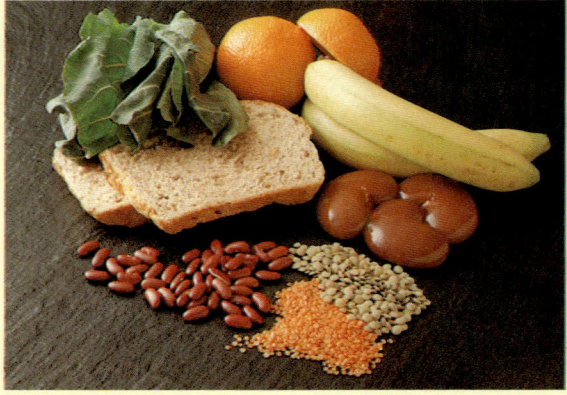

FOLIC ACID helps fight anaemia, which can arise in pregnancy from a deficiency of folic acid. Main sources: offal, raw dark green leafy vegetables, pulses, wholemeal bread, oranges, bananas. Your doctor may prescribe folic acid in tablet form.

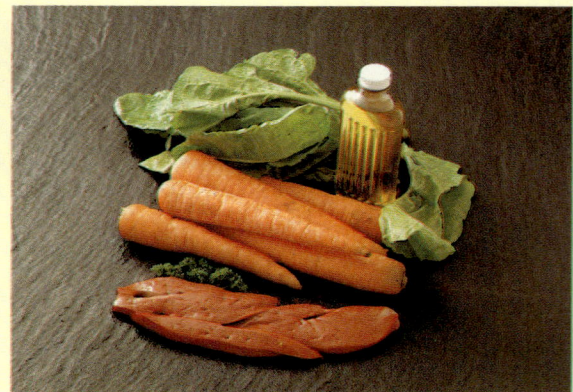

VITAMIN A builds up your resistance to infection and will also help relieve allergies and maintain healthy skin. Main sources: liver, halibut liver oil, carrots, spinach, also milk and butter.

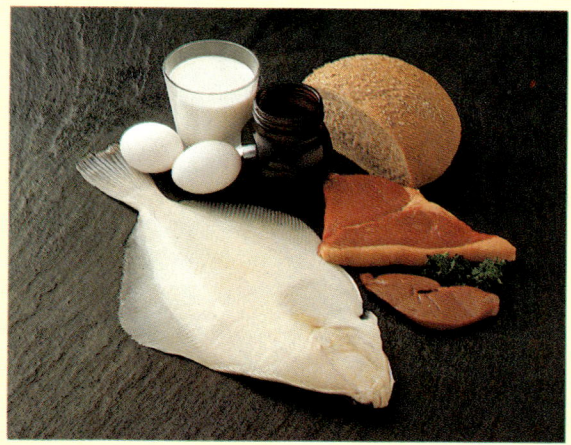

B VITAMINS are important for many different body functions. They are essential for a healthy skin, for mental stability, and for the proper functioning of the digestive system. After the birth they increase the production of milk for breastfeeding. Main sources: meat, liver, milk, eggs, wholemeal bread, wheatgerm, fish, yeast extract.

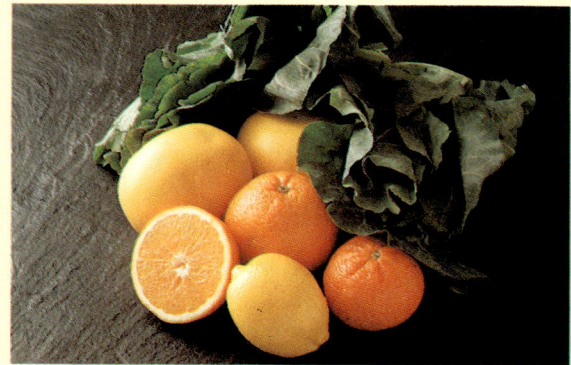

VITAMIN C helps the body absorb iron and keeps the tissues strong and healthy. Main sources: citrus fruit, green vegetables.

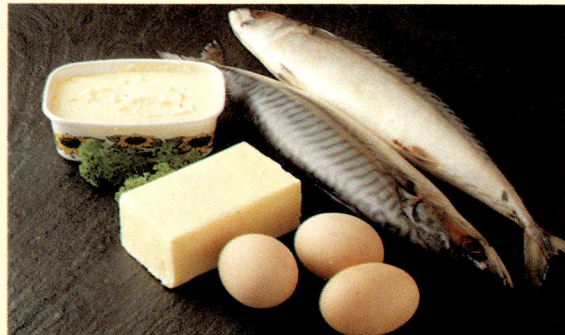

VITAMIN D aids the body in maintaining the level of calcium and phosphorus in the blood. Main sources: fatty fish, eggs, butter, margarine. It is also produced when the body is exposed to sunlight.

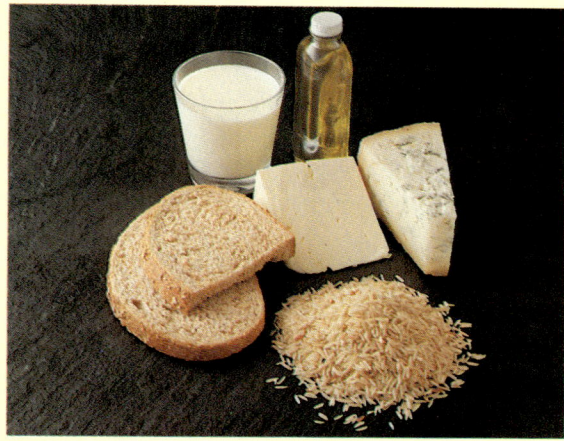

VITAMIN E can help strengthen the foetus and placenta, and improve the circulation thus preventing varicose veins and piles. Main sources: eggs, dairy products, unpolished rice, wholemeal bread, vegetable oils. Vitamin E supplement (wheatgerm oil) can be bought from a chemist or health food shop. You should never take vitamin E and iron together as the effectiveness of vitamin E is destroyed by iron – a twelve hour gap between them is necessary to avoid this.

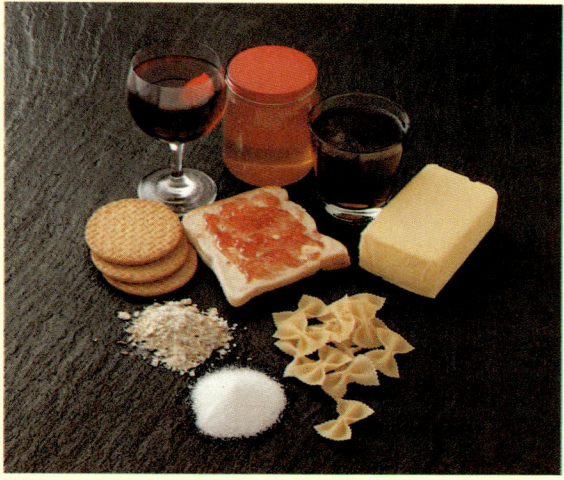

FATS AND CARBOHYDRATES provide energy and build up reserves of body fat. They also contain fat-soluble vitamins and minerals. Main sources of fats: butter, margarine, fatty meat and oily fish, dairy products. Main sources of unrefined carbohydrates: wholemeal bread, cereals, pasta, brown rice, potatoes, fruit. These are an essential part of a balanced diet. Main sources of refined carbohydrate (not good for you): sugar, cakes, biscuits, sweets, jam, soft drinks and alcohol.

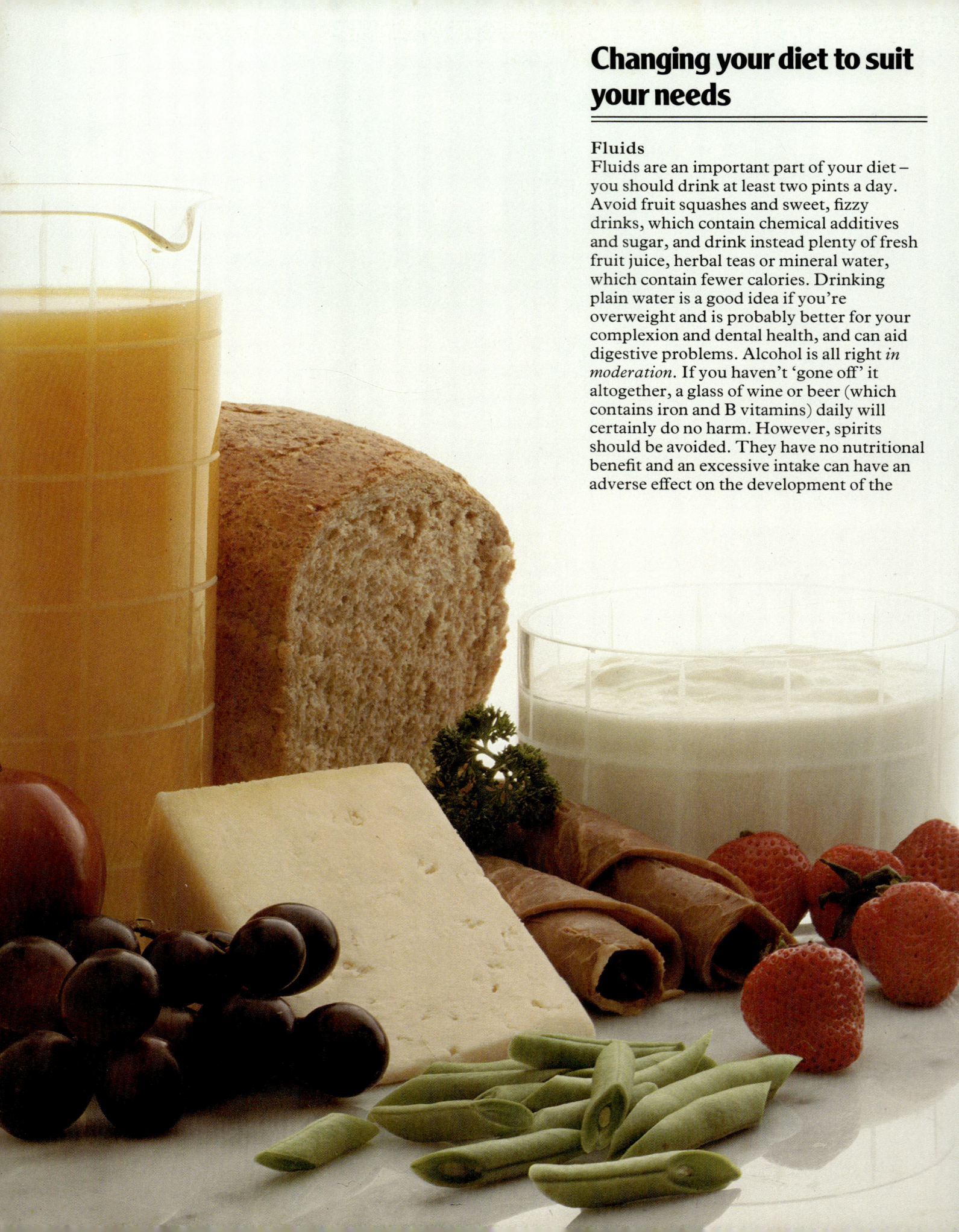

Changing your diet to suit your needs

Fluids

Fluids are an important part of your diet – you should drink at least two pints a day. Avoid fruit squashes and sweet, fizzy drinks, which contain chemical additives and sugar, and drink instead plenty of fresh fruit juice, herbal teas or mineral water, which contain fewer calories. Drinking plain water is a good idea if you're overweight and is probably better for your complexion and dental health, and can aid digestive problems. Alcohol is all right *in moderation*. If you haven't 'gone off' it altogether, a glass of wine or beer (which contains iron and B vitamins) daily will certainly do no harm. However, spirits should be avoided. They have no nutritional benefit and an excessive intake can have an adverse effect on the development of the baby, making it less active in the womb than it should be.

Vegetarians and vegans
Vegetarians and vegans should take extra care that they are getting enough protein in their daily diet, since it is an essential body-building material for both mother and child. For vegetarians, cheese, eggs and milk are the prime sources of protein, for vegans, other good sources are green vegetables, dried fruits, pulses (dried beans, lentils, etc.), nuts and seeds, wholemeal bread and cereals.

If you don't eat dairy produce it is particularly important that you eat as many protein-enriched foods as possible to get the right balance of proteins. Soya bean is an almost perfect substitute for animal protein and there is a variety of soya products – soya milk, soya flour and soya meat (TVP). Pasta, muesli, lentils, wheatgerm and all nuts are further good sources. It is also advisable to take vitamin B supplement since these vitamins and especially B_{12} are found mainly in animal foods – yeast extract is a good source. Some women may feel that they prefer not to take iron or folic acid in tablet form but if you are a vegetarian or vegan, it is safer not to rely on diet alone during pregnancy. If you are determined to keep up your iron intake through diet however, soya, treacle and cocoa powder are valuable sources. Folic acid is present in raw dark green leafy vegetables but is readily destroyed by cooking.

Constipation
Pregnant women are more prone to constipation, as the hormone that relaxes ligaments and muscles during pregnancy also tends to relax the bowel muscles. This problem can be helped by eating high-fibre food such as bran cereals, wholemeal bread, figs, fresh fruit and vegetables. It is also important to make sure you are drinking enough. If you still find constipation a problem don't be tempted to take a laxative without asking the doctor first. He will almost certainly recommend an alkali preparation or a senna derivative, but these should be used only when absolutely necessary and really, although it would be ideal to open the bowels once a day, it is not imperative providing you always spare the time to do so when nature calls. Hurrying and straining will inevitably result in piles.

Piles or haemorrhoids are varicose veins in and around the rectum – the pressure of the uterus on the anal canal can enlarge the veins and straining to empty the bowel just aggravates matters. Piles usually start off as an irritation around the anus and if they are not treated with an ointment prescribed by a doctor they may bleed and become very painful indeed.

Heartburn and Indigestion
At some time during your pregnancy – usually after the thirtieth week – you may suffer from heartburn and indigestion. This is due to acidity from the stomach being forced up into the gullet by the enlarging uterus. Eating a lot will make this feeling worse and your appetite may diminish considerably. Avoid large meals, particularly before bed, fried or spicy foods and alcohol, chocolate, orange juice or coffee. Smaller meals eaten more frequently should help, because if you allow too great a gap between meals your stomach may empty completely, probably causing heartburn. Try sucking strong minty sweets (clean your teeth regularly if you do this) and avoid lying flat at night, slumping or bending too far forward. If the problem persists consult your doctor who will probably prescribe an antacid mixture.

Cravings
Pregnant women can be most unpredictable in their choice of food – especially during the first three months of pregnancy. Your tastes alter – sometimes dramatically – due to the hormonal, metabolic and chemical changes going on in your body. During pregnancy some women develop strong desires for foods they never particularly liked before and wouldn't normally think of eating. There are old stories of pregnant women eating soil and even digging for coal. A really abnormal desire like this is called *pica* (the Latin word for magpie – a bird that collects strange things) and has been interpreted as a subconscious urge to supplement a nutritional deficiency with essential minerals. *Pica* is uncommon today now that most people are more nutritionally aware and iron and vitamin tablets are readily available.

Quirky food cravings are usually physiological and there are some foods that are high in certain sources of nourishment and all the better for you should you develop a sudden passion for them. Some odd cravings reported are for black pudding (high in iron), pilchards (full of calcium, protein and iron), and nuts (rich in mineral salts, protein and fats). It is very common to have a craving for carbohydrate foods, which may be related to a high demand for glucose by the placenta.

Morning sickness

This is a classic symptom of pregnancy and can range from a sensation of queasiness to actual vomiting. Try and relieve this by eating a couple of dry biscuits, a slice of toast or by sucking acid drops, mints or boiled sweets before you attempt to get out of bed. Even if you are not actually sick you may well suffer some degree of nausea and this can persist throughout the day and evening accompanied by a strange metallic or greasy taste in the mouth. Ironically you may find that eating relieves the nausea, so it is often helpful to take constant small snacks rather than tackle a large plate of food. The most comforting snacks are usually the starchy ones. If anything upsets you – the strong smell of brewing coffee or the greasiness of frying are common irritants – avoid it. Even if you really feel that you can't eat anything, do try to get down something small, starchy and light as often as you can manage.

If you are a smoker you may find that cigarettes become distasteful. Take this ideal opportunity to give them up for good. If you haven't gone off smoking, doctors do advise that you should try to stop anyway. Evidence has shown that the oxygen supply to the baby through the placenta is reduced by smoking, which increases the risk of abortion or premature birth and can result in smaller and less intelligent children. If you really cannot stop, try to cut down to seven or fewer a day.

Thankfully, the symptoms of nausea almost always pass off by the twelfth to fourteenth week of pregnancy when the level of the hormone chorionic gonadotrophin (the hormone that is initially responsible for the continuance of pregnancy) drops, and your appetite returns to normal.

The anti-nausea meal plan

If you feel sick or nauseous all day you will probably find that frequent snacks help alleviate the discomfort. It is mainly carbohydrate foods that do the trick and although eating citrus fruits, apples or raw carrots may help slightly, it's generally the bland and starchy foods that are most effective. If you fancy toast, butter it lightly. Plain biscuits are better for you than sweet ones. Thick soups are filling yet gentle on the stomach. If drinking with your meals makes you feel sick, try to drink between them – you might find cold drinks more palatable than hot milky drinks, which are not particularly thirst-quenching. If your stomach cannot tolerate milky drinks, then

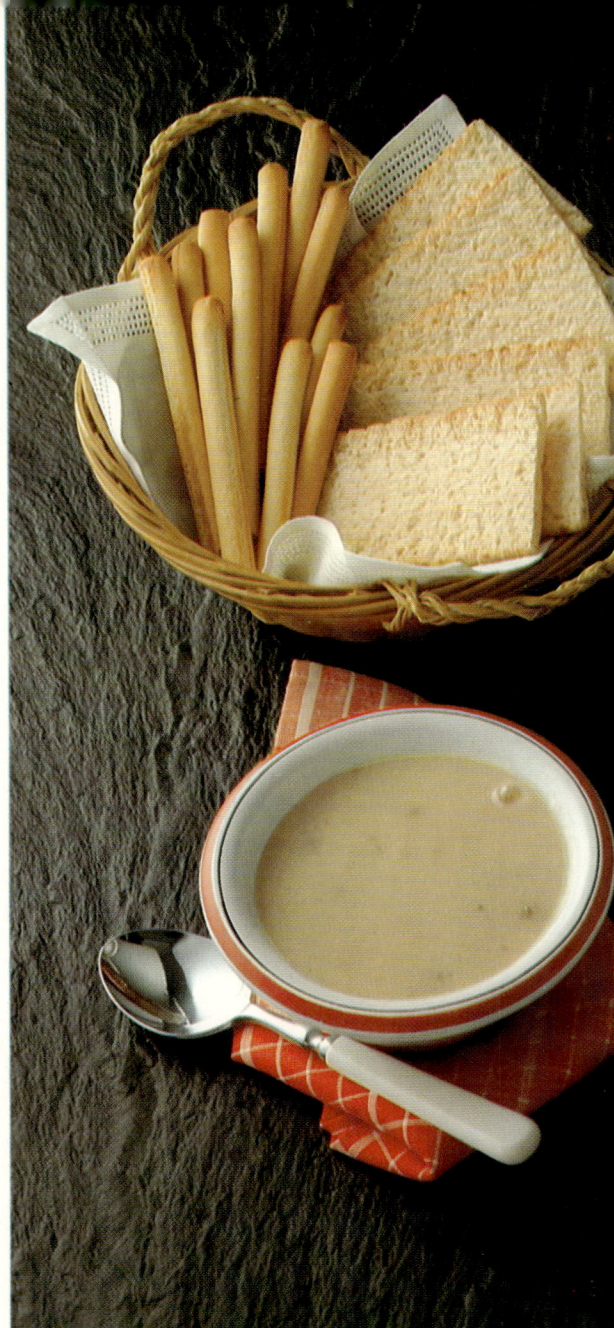

fruit juices, glucose and soda drinks, such as Lucozade, lemonade and mineral water make good substitutes. All the foods below should be taken in small amounts, very frequently, until the sickness goes. Providing you don't over-eat you won't put on extra weight.

ON WAKING

Semi-sweet biscuits or dry cracker or toast
Small sips of a sweetened drink

BREAKFAST

A small amount of cereal or porridge or stewed apples or prunes
Toast with marmalade, jam or honey

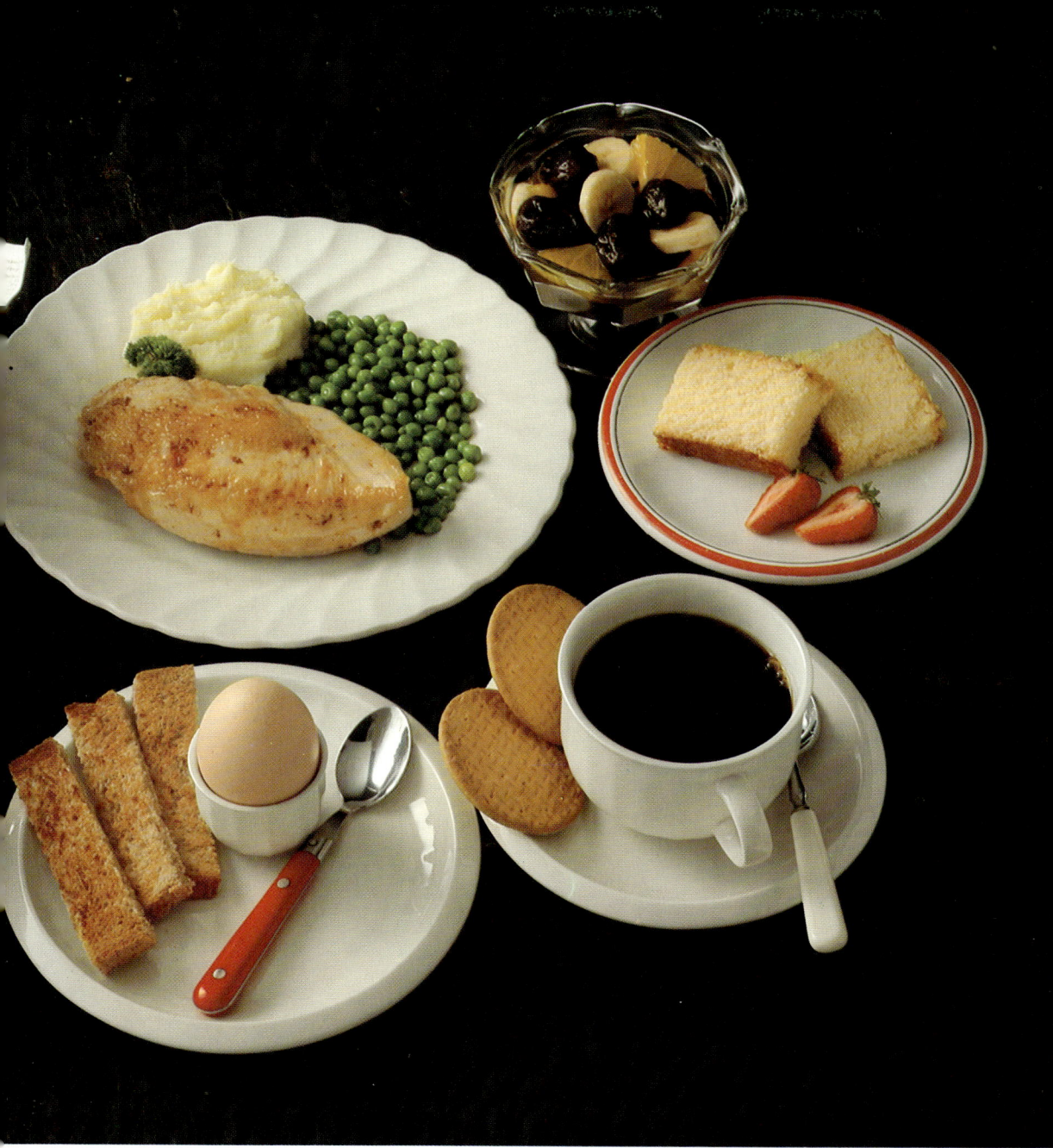

Eating little and often is the answer for nausea and morning sickness, frequent small snacks of mainly bland starchy foods being the most effective way to relieve these classic symptoms of pregnancy.

MORNING SNACK

Dry toast, cracker or biscuit
Fresh fruit

LUNCH

Cream soup or boiled egg
Bread, toast or cracker
Egg custard or ice cream or fresh or stewed fruit

AFTERNOON SNACK

Fresh fruit, toast or biscuit

TEA

Dry toast with jam or honey
Biscuit or piece of sponge cake

SUPPER

Cream soup
Mashed potato and vegetables, e.g. carrots, peas, with a small portion of fish or chicken if desired
Rice pudding or fruit or raisins or a piece of cake or a biscuit

EVENING SNACK

Dry toast, biscuit or cracker

BEDTIME

Two slices dry toast, two biscuits or cereal

NIGHT

Keep dry biscuits and a drink by your bed

Have a small drink with each snack or between snacks, whichever suits you best.

Skin and Make-up

Many pregnant women acquire a definite bloom to their complexion as pregnancy advances beyond the first twelve weeks and any feelings of nausea and sickness subside. In fact, this rosy glow is due mainly to extra blood circulating around the body. By the thirty-fourth week of pregnancy the amount of blood in the circulation may have increased by as much as fifty per cent and remains virtually the same until the birth, when hormone levels fall and the body goes back to its non-pregnant state.

On the whole, pregnant women find that their skin condition changes during pregnancy – usually for the better. This may be because of the increased blood flow to the skin or possibly because they are eating more sensibly or taking life at a slower pace and therefore are less susceptible to stress. Dry skins tend to become oilier and more supple, oily skins may become drier (although the reverse may also be true). Some women do find that spots appear unexpectedly; this is probably due to the action of progesterone, which increases sebaceous activity. Cleanse the skin thoroughly every night and try to eat more fresh fruit and vegetables rather than chocolate and fatty foods (see page 42 for which vitamins affect your skin). If, however, you continue to have problems with your skin and nothing seems to work, your doctor may refer you to a dermatologist.

Some rounding of the face is normal during pregnancy – a plumpness of the cheeks and beneath the jaw is due to fluid retention and extra fat deposits. While the face should not become really swollen – a condition associated with excessive fluid retention – that slight extra fullness will help to plump out lines and wrinkles making you look younger and healthier.

Skin care-a daily routine

Even though your complexion may have improved during pregnancy, it is still important to keep your skin clean, and not to neglect it. It is only necessary to cleanse the skin once a day but it must be done thoroughly and gently. Start with the eyes. If you wear a waterproof mascara you will need an oil-based product to remove it,

otherwise a non-oily eye make-up remover is effective. When cleansing the eyes, never scrub – use balls of dampened cotton wool and stroke gently from the brow downwards. Always work from the outer corner to the inner corner underneath the bottom lashes – that way you won't stretch the delicate skin.

Bad handling of your skin can do as much harm as neglecting it. The best cleanser for every skin type is a liquid, milky lotion, which should be applied to your face with the fingertips and wiped off. Repeat this several times, making sure that all dirt and grime have been removed and that the last tissue you use is clean after wiping the skin. If you wash your face after using a cleansing lotion it is probably best not to use soap, as it can be very drying. Instead, use a wash cleanser, which comes in liquid or granule form – or a soap-free cleansing bar. First wet your face with lukewarm water, then rub a small amount of cleanser gently on to your damp skin with the fingertips. Rinse off well. Don't use a flannel or sponge on your face if you have spots – they are a breeding ground for germs. For the same

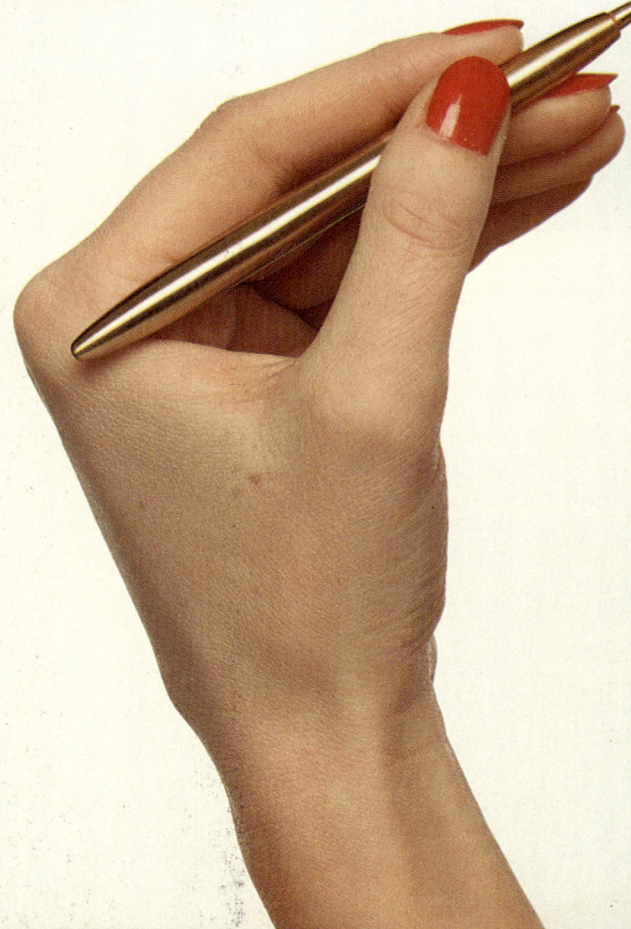

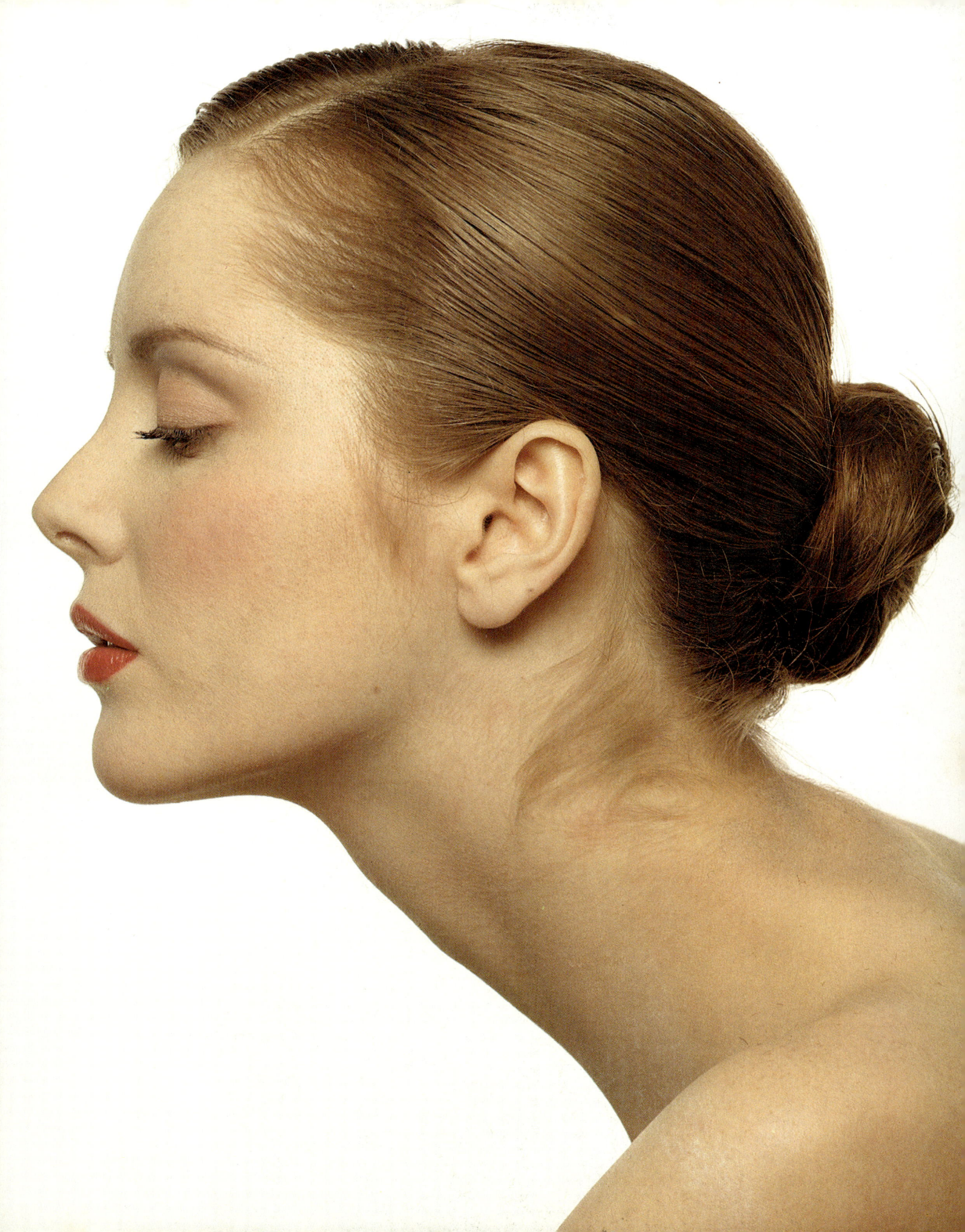

reason, dry your face with paper towels.

Toning is especially important if you have developed spots, as it will remove any last traces of make-up and the alcohol in it will have an antiseptic action. A mild toner or freshener – that is, one without alcohol – is best if you have dry skin. If you find that the toner you are using is too strong and stings, dilute it with pure rosewater – available from a chemist's dispensary. Apply toner on cotton wool that has been dampened and wrung out; this will make it less concentrated and ensure that it goes further.

A skin that has become dry may flake and become itchy and also tends to emphasize wrinkles. So if your skin feels very dry use a moisturizing cream during the day (always apply moisturizer to a slightly damp skin), and also a night cream, to prevent water loss and replace oils. Pay particular attention to the delicate skin around the eyes and mouth – there are special eye creams available. In fact it's probably more likely that your skin will become greasier, in which case you won't need a night cream. However, a moisturizer worn during the day acts as a protective layer between your skin and your make-up and so is advisable whatever your skin type, but make sure that it is water-based if you have an oily skin.

A natural make-up

During pregnancy you want to enhance the new glow in order to focus attention on your face and not on the bulge. But don't overdo it, a natural make-up is best at this time (you may look younger anyway as the cheeks plump out); anything startling or outrageous can look absurd.

Foundation
Choose a foundation that matches your natural skin colour, taking the tone from your neck. This may seem a little pale, but a blusher should give colour, not foundation. Use the back of your hand as a palette (so that you don't put too much on at once) and with your fingertips or a sponge apply the foundation to your face in sections, starting with the cheeks and forehead. Stroke downwards in the direction of the hairs of the face or you will tend to get a matted look. Stipple a little extra foundation over broken veins or blemishes – a natural look is achieved by applying many thin layers rather than one thick one.

Use an eye stick or under-eye cover cream in a lighter shade than your foundation to conceal any dark shadows under the eyes. Again warm and thin it on the back of the hand first. Don't rub the stick under your eye or it will drag the delicate skin.

Blusher
If you like to wear a blusher, powder is easier to use than a cream or gel. A pinky tone will look most natural, particularly if you have a high colour or broken veins, since it won't clash with pink cheeks or a sudden flush. Fill the blusher brush with powder, tapping off the excess. Smile, and apply to the cheekbones just below the middle of the eye and outwards towards the hairline.

Powder
Use a translucent loose powder to set your make-up – it needn't look powdery and does help make-up last longer. Don't use a coloured powder on top of a coloured foundation: as your face warms up oils are

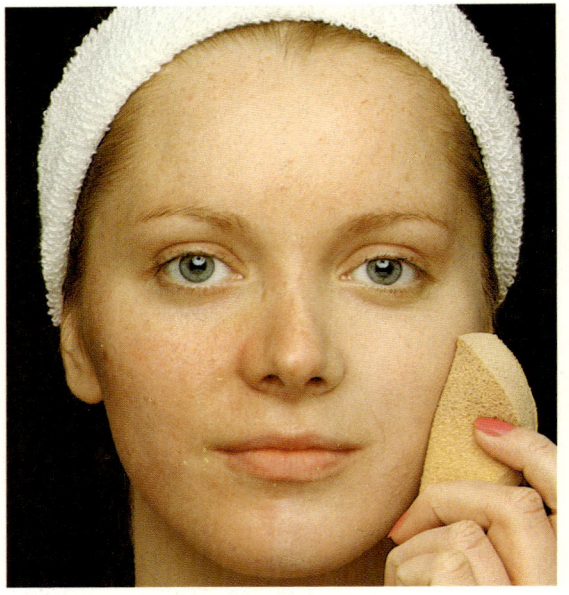

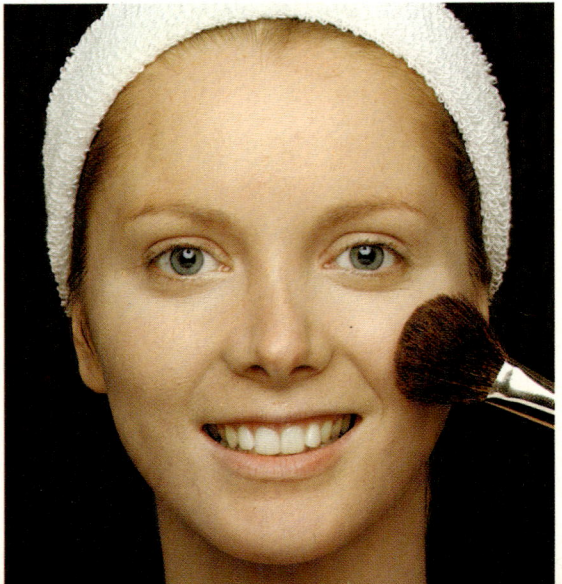

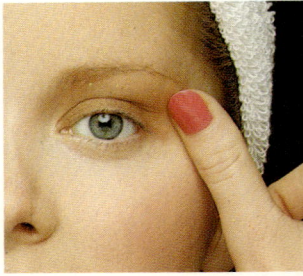

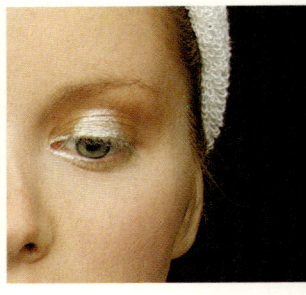

Left: match your foundation to your natural skin colour, taking the tone from your neck, and then brush on a pinky blusher to bring some colour to your cheeks.

Centre: Soft colours are the most flattering for eyes. Fade the shadow out towards the eyebrow and then highlight the centre of the lid and inner corner of the eye with white frosty shadow to add a little sparkle.

Right: Fair people can emphasize their eyes with a very fine line of dark liner drawn at the base of the upper lashes. Similarly, the shape of the mouth is better defined by outlining the top lip with white frosty shadow before applying lip colour.

released that may cause the two colour pigments to react on one another and change – and you could end up with an orange face. Shake some powder on to a wodge of cotton wool and press on to the skin. Do not scrub and scrape or your carefully placed make-up will be moved. Turn the cotton wool over and flick any excess powder off the face.

The eyes

Bright hard colours will kill the colour of your eyes and their natural sparkle, so choose soft sludgy browns, greys, and mauves to set them off. Blue and green are hard colours but their effect is softened if used in conjunction with brown, grey or mauve.

Apply eye shadow all over the eye area from lashes to eyebrow, but fade it out towards the eyebrow and blend well at the edges.

To give extra sparkle to your eyes, take a white frosty shadow and draw a white triangle on the centre of the upper lid, and then outline with a 'V' the innermost corner of each eye. If your lashes are very fair you may find it useful to have them dyed regularly, so that the roots always look dark. Otherwise you can emphasize them by drawing a *very* fine line right at the base of the upper lashes with dark liner, carefully using the edge of the brush.

To achieve a natural silky look to the eyelashes, apply several thin coats of mascara and always wipe the brush on a tissue first to blot off any excess mascara that would clog up the lashes.

Lip colour

Choose soft lip colours to go with your clothes. Glossy colours accentuate small lips, use flatter colours for large lips. Lines drawn round the lips first with a brush will help to define the shape of the mouth, or outline the top lip only with a white frosty shadow (the same one you have used for your eyes), as we show here.

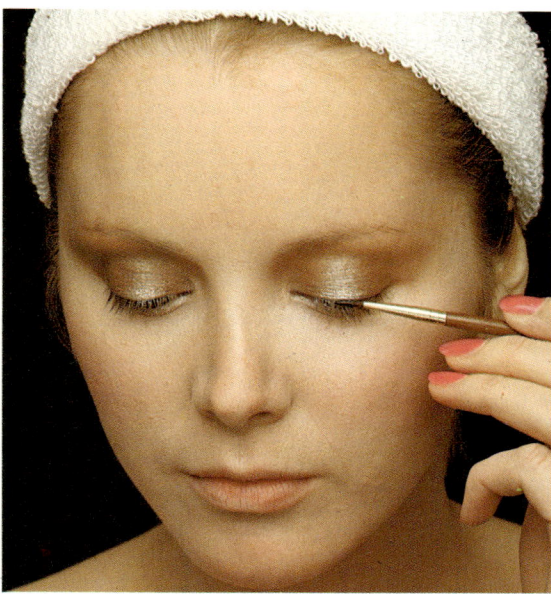

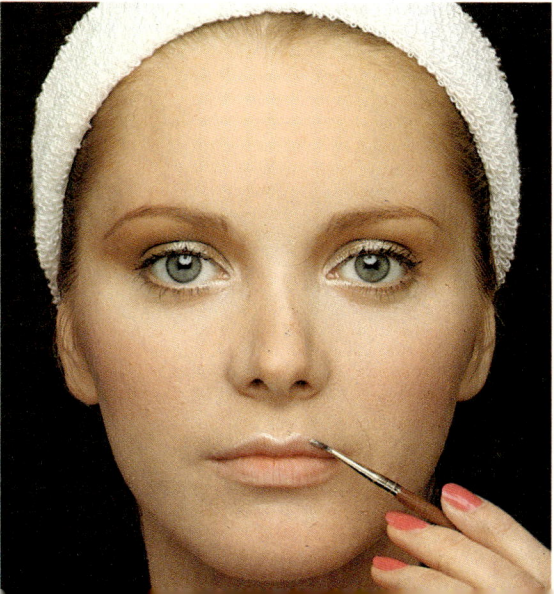

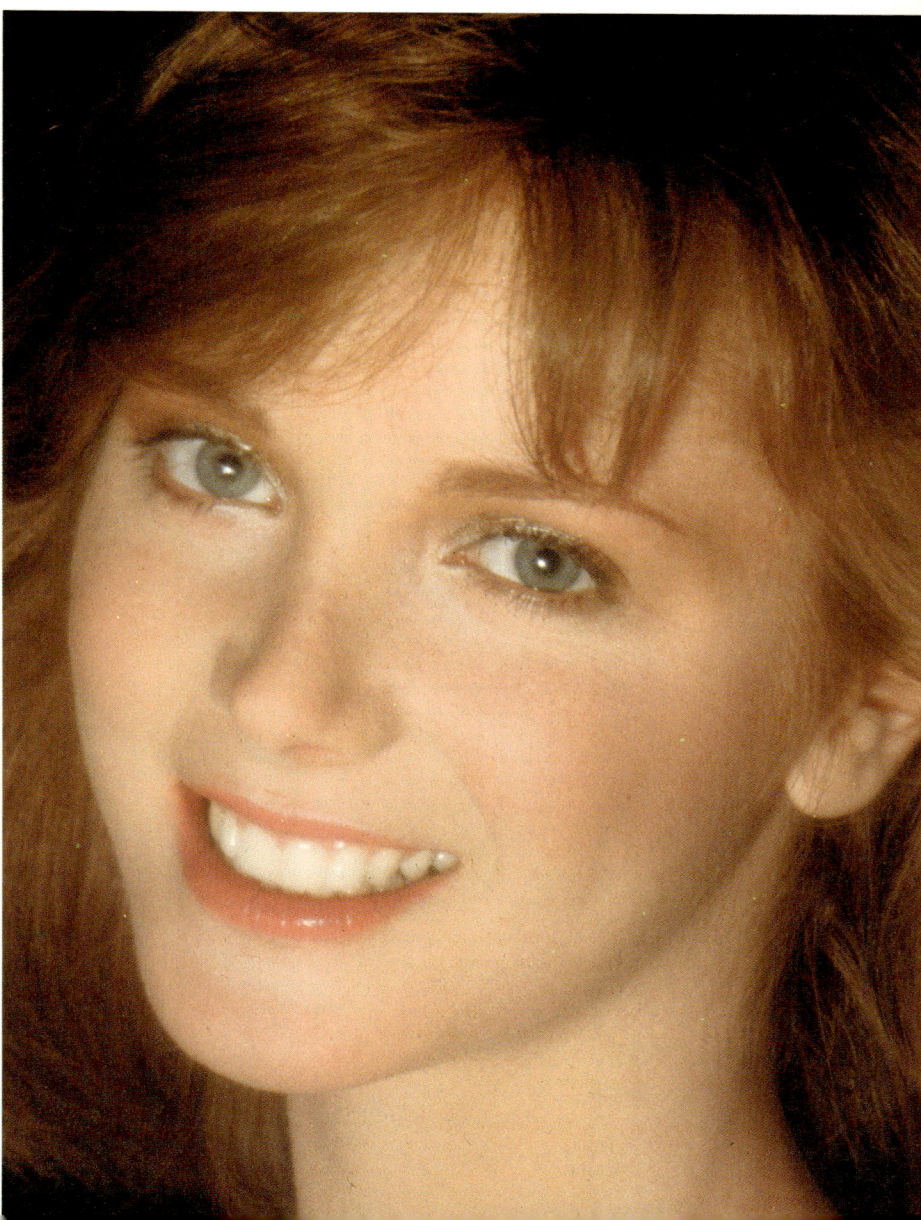

Camouflage make-up

If at any time during pregnancy the 'bloom' seems to elude you and you find that your face has become puffy, or that hormonal changes or bad sleeping habits are causing skin problems, there are ways to camouflage these bad points and to minimize their effect on your appearance.

Dark circles under the eyes
Dark circles may be emphasized by tiredness during pregnancy. To disguise the dark area, use a good under-eye cover cream that is fine in texture. Rub a small amount between your thumb and finger to warm and thin it before stippling it on with your fingers over a thin layer of foundation. Cover with another thin layer of foundation and blend carefully.

Puffiness or bags under the eyes
Fluid retention during pregnancy can cause this puffiness, which again is increased by tiredness and strain. Use a good eye mask while resting to reduce the puffiness (cucumber slices are also very good for this). To camouflage, use a very fine eyeliner brush to paint a light-coloured under-eye cover cream along the dark line underneath the 'bag'. The light shade will bring the dark line forward; do not apply it to the puffy area or this will appear to be even more prominent. Blend in carefully and cover with foundation.

Pink Eyes
Tiredness or the increased blood in the circulation may make your eyes look bloodshot. Use a gentle eye mask to soothe them while you are resting and safe eye drops to bring back a little sparkle.

Greasy or dry patches
Pregnancy may cause your skin to become greasier or drier than usual. Greasiness is more likely because of the action of progesterone. For greasy patches use only a water-based moisturizer and a fine-textured, non-oil based foundation and translucent powder. For dry patches you need an oil-based moisturizer and a sparing amount of foundation and powder. If the skin is flaking use no foundation or powder at all as these will only show up the problem.

Wrinkles and crows feet
During early pregnancy the skin may become drier than usual, which can make fine lines and wrinkles more apparent. Use a very fine-textured foundation over the problem area and only the finest translucent powder – anything heavy or containing a shine will accentuate the wrinkles. Anti-wrinkle creams can temporarily disguise wrinkles by charging the skin with fluid, but certainly won't cure them.

Spots
A change in the hormone balance can produce spots. As long as you cleanse properly, water-based make-up will not make spots worse (though note that anything with an oil, lanolin or paraffin base probably will) so there is no reason why you shouldn't use it to conceal them. If they are not too bad just stipple a little extra foundation over the spots with a brush or your finger. If this is not sufficient, apply water-based foundation and then stipple with a spot-erase stick or cream in the same shade. Finish with another stipple of foundation, and then translucent powder.

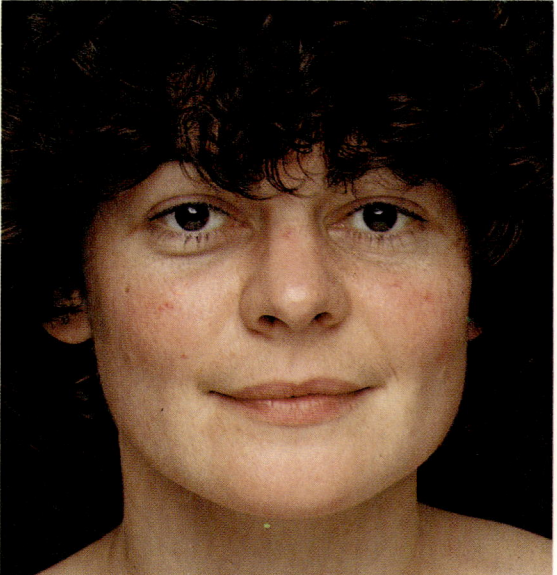

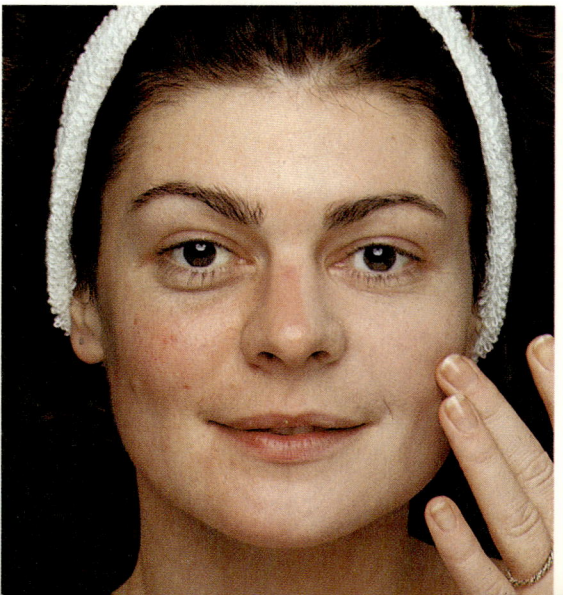

Left: Choose a flat, beige foundation to cover over-pink cheeks and broken veins, applying several thin layers rather than one thick one.

Centre: If you suffer from puffiness or bags under the eyes, a light-coloured under-eye cover cream painted along the dark line beneath the bag will make this less evident, while safe eye drops will help to restore the sparkle to tired eyes.

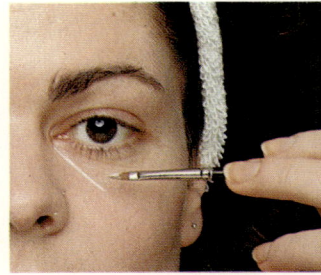

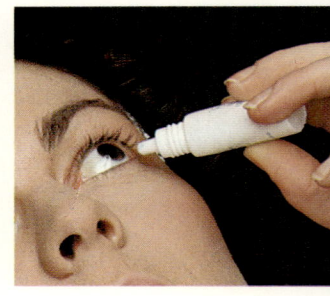

Right: Spots can be concealed with a stipple of spot-erase stick or cream over your usual foundation, and the classic puffiness under the chin camouflaged by brushing a browny shader beneath the jawline.

Puffiness under the chin

Puffiness under the chin is probably more likely to occur later on in pregnancy and is again due to fluid retention. Camouflage by subtle shading with a browny shade of blusher or shader. Brush this under the jawline and on either side of the neck. Use the same blusher to emphasize your cheekbones – feel for the bone and then brush up on to it with a flicking movement. Use a pinky blusher on the temples to bring the attention to your eyes and away from the jawline.

High colour in the cheeks

The extra blood circulating is responsible for your 'bloom' and an increased metabolic rate may make you feel more heated. To tone down very pink cheeks, use a flat, beige foundation (there should be no hint of pink in it) that is not too thick or greasy – or it will separate on your skin – and apply it in two or three very thin layers, stippling on extra where needed. Green foundation is sometimes advocated for concealing high colour and you could try this under your usual foundation, but it may just make you look green and ghostly. The idea originated from the theatre where the green counteracted the red in the bright lights.

Pigmentation on the face

Brunettes especially may notice increased pigmentation of the face – freckles, birthmarks and moles may get darker especially after exposure to the sun. Sometimes the sun will bring out a butterfly-shaped 'mask' over the cheeks, nose and forehead (see page 26). This can be camouflaged with an erase stick blended with foundation. Never attempt to bleach.

Dry lips

Breathing through the mouth because of a blocked-up nose during pregnancy may cause one to lick the lips a lot, which can make them very dry. Rub in vaseline and camouflage with a glossy lipstick.

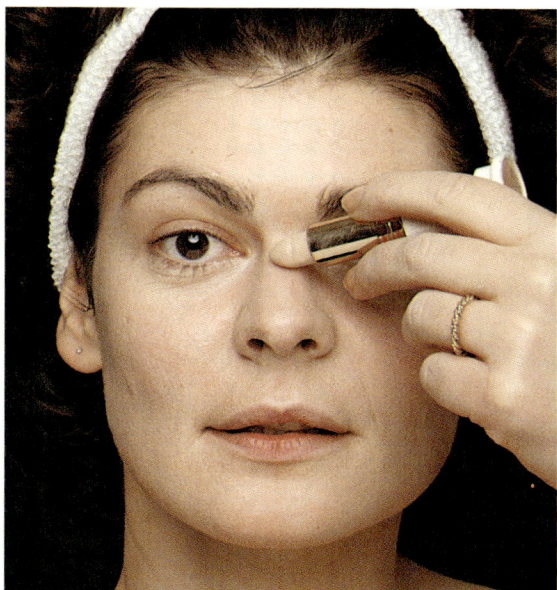

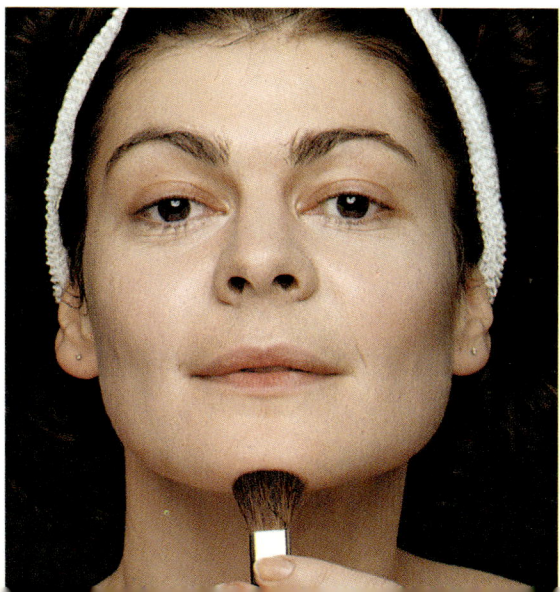

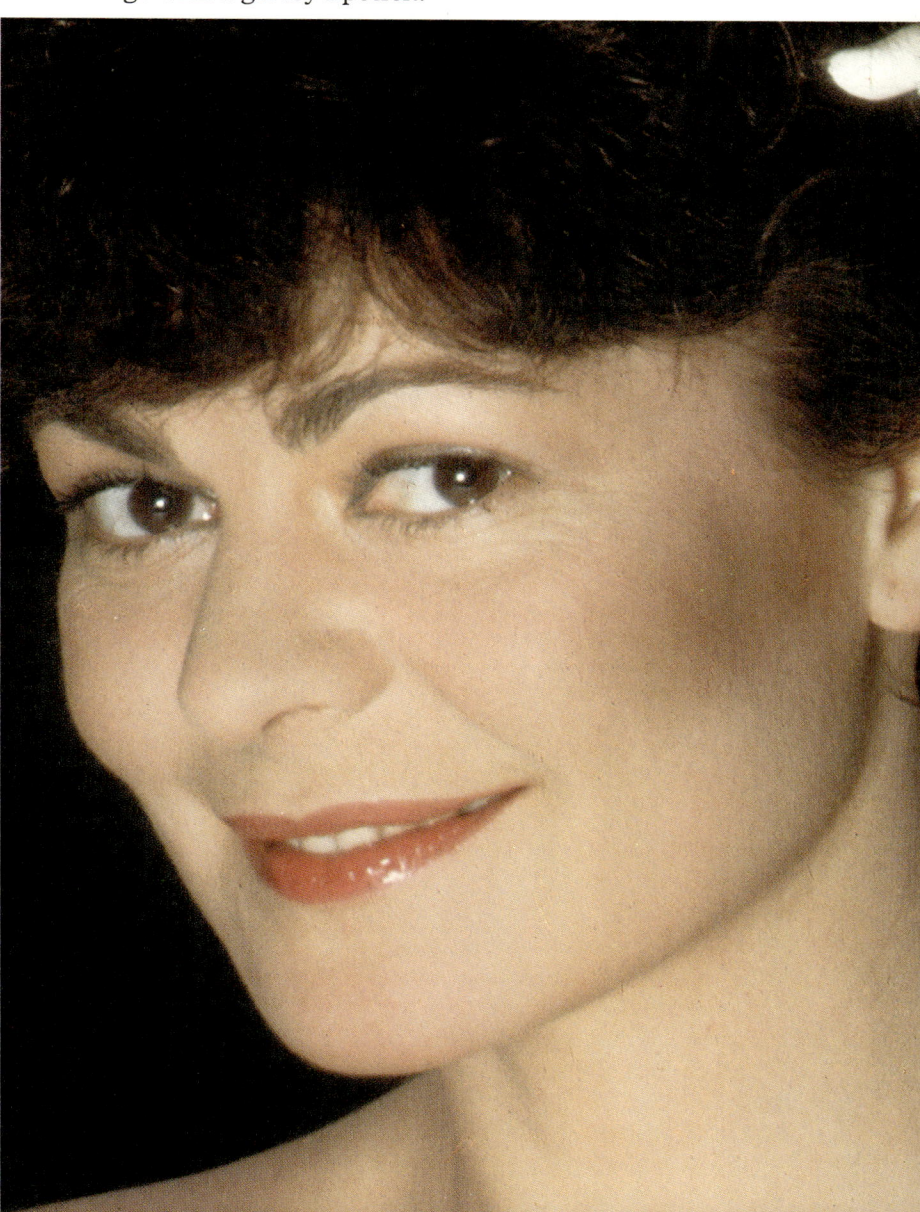

Hair

With all the upheavals going on in your body it is inevitable that the condition of your hair will change to some extent – whether for better or for worse. But while the re-balancing of hormones is undoubtedly responsible for this, the state of your health also has a lot to do with it and some trichologists feel that the best hair tonic of all comes from a pregnant woman's own effort and well-being. For instance, you are probably taking more interest in your diet, making sure you get the right vitamins and so on. You may have stopped smoking or at least cut down. You probably don't drink as much alcohol as before. You are possibly taking life a little slower and sitting with your feet up more often and are therefore more relaxed. So, although nature plays a large part in your appearance during pregnancy, so does the way you look after yourself.

Many women find that their hair in fact changes for the better during pregnancy even though it does tend to become a little greasier. This is because the body is producing extra sebum (or oil) which protects the elasticity and prevents the hair from splitting. You may need to wash your hair more often but if you use a mild shampoo you should have a healthy, shining head of hair.

If, on the other hand, your hair seems to have become drier (less sebum) take extra care. It may break more easily and because of this more may fall out than usual. In this case, use a very mild shampoo and be careful not to brush or comb your hair harshly or to use too much heat on it when drying – rather let it dry naturally. If the condition of your hair has not improved after the first twelve weeks or so – or indeed has deteriorated – it is probably not the fault of your pregnancy at all. Perhaps you are not in particularly good health. Try to include more fresh fruit and vegetables in your diet and see your doctor if you feel very run down. You may be worrying or feeling tense or may not be getting enough rest. If you have tried to remedy your hair problem without success think about how you feel in yourself and don't be afraid to discuss this with your doctor.

The increase in metabolic activity during pregnancy causes a greater amount of blood than usual to reach the skin and you may find that you often feel hot and sweaty.

Because you sweat more frequently your hair may well become lank towards the end of pregnancy. The only answer here is frequent washing to keep it looking fresh and clean. This will not do your hair any harm, but always use a mild baby shampoo or a herbal shampoo to avoid stripping off the natural oils.

Hair grows much faster during pregnancy than at any other time but this rapid growth rate slows down after the birth. Some women find that a considerable amount of hair actually falls out after delivery, which can be worrying. However, this is a perfectly normal thing to happen and it will certainly not lead to baldness – new hair begins to grow in to replace the hair that has been lost almost immediately.

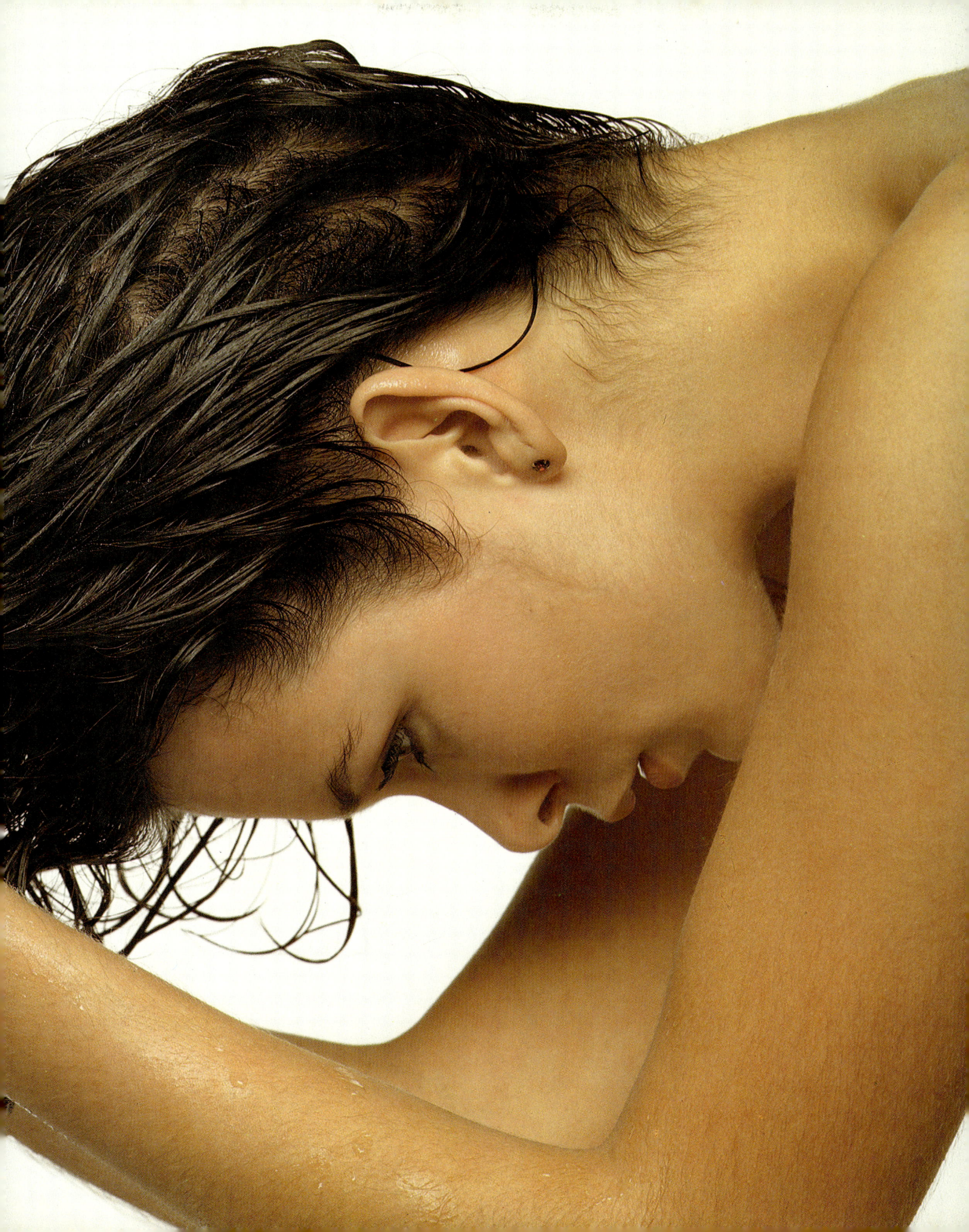

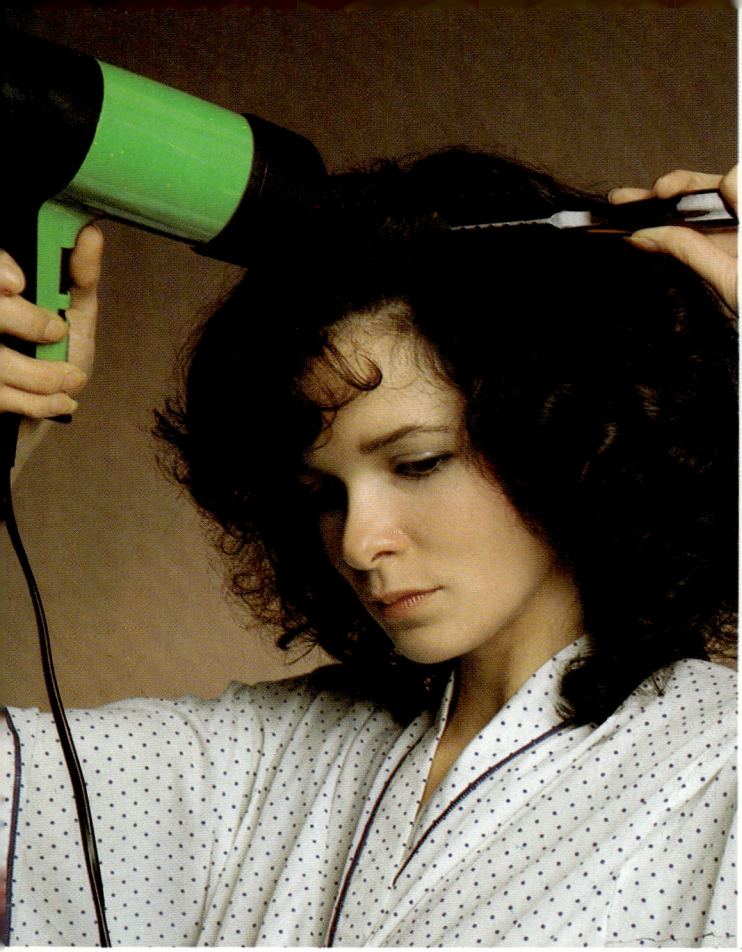

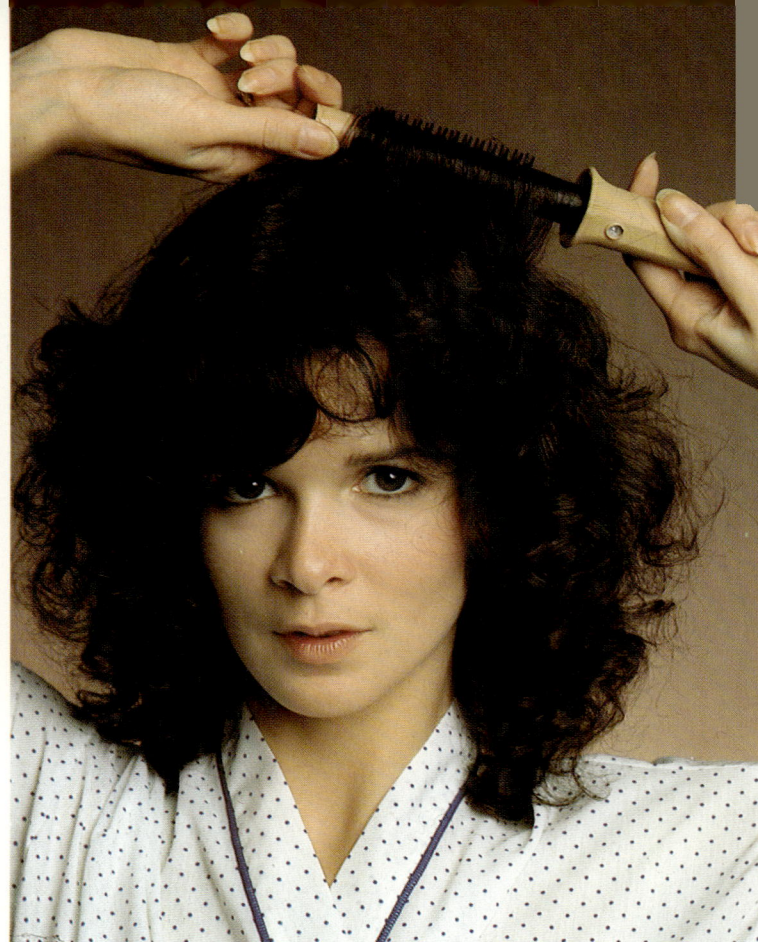

Sit comfortably on a straight-backed chair when using a hair dryer or curling tongs and be careful not to overheat your hair.

At the hairdresser

A good cut is an asset; not only will it make looking after your hair a great deal easier, it should also help balance the shape of your head with the changing shape of your body. For instance, a cropped hair cut could make your head look awfully small in comparison to the rest of you and maybe a fuller hairstyle would be more flattering. In the following pages we have suggested styles for different face shapes – including ones that have filled out and become more rounded – and different types of hair.

But what about perming and colouring? Some hairdressers prefer not to use chemical colourants on a woman's hair during pregnancy as there is a risk of the dyes entering the bloodstream via a tiny nick or scratch on the scalp. It has not been proved that they could be harmful to the baby but some doctors advise against using hair products that contain potent chemical dyes. Vegetable colourings such as henna and camomile are harmless and probably far better for the condition of your hair under these circumstances.

There is a theory that the ammonia fumes from a perm may possibly affect the baby via your blood – although there is no evidence to support this. Generally doctors do not advise against perming or bleaching after the first three months. Many trichologists maintain that with the increased amount of elasticity that the hair has at this time, there is no reason why a perm should not take and be most effective. However, a hairdresser is often over-cautious if a client is pregnant, and tends to under-process the hair. Either he takes the solution off too soon or doesn't make it strong enough. Hence the perm doesn't take – not harmful, but a total waste of money. Always discuss these aspects with your hairdresser before you go ahead. The best time for a perm is around the twenty-fourth to the twenty-sixth week of pregnancy. Your hair should then be in peak condition and the perm will last until well after the baby is born.

If you are having problems with dry hair, though, you should probably decide against having a perm as this will inevitably dry out the hair further, making it even more prone to splitting and breaking. If the condition of your hair isn't tip-top (through ill-health or too much perming, bleaching and colouring) it is best to avoid causing more havoc.

Haircare at home

Although in early pregnancy nausea and sickness may not make you feel disposed to

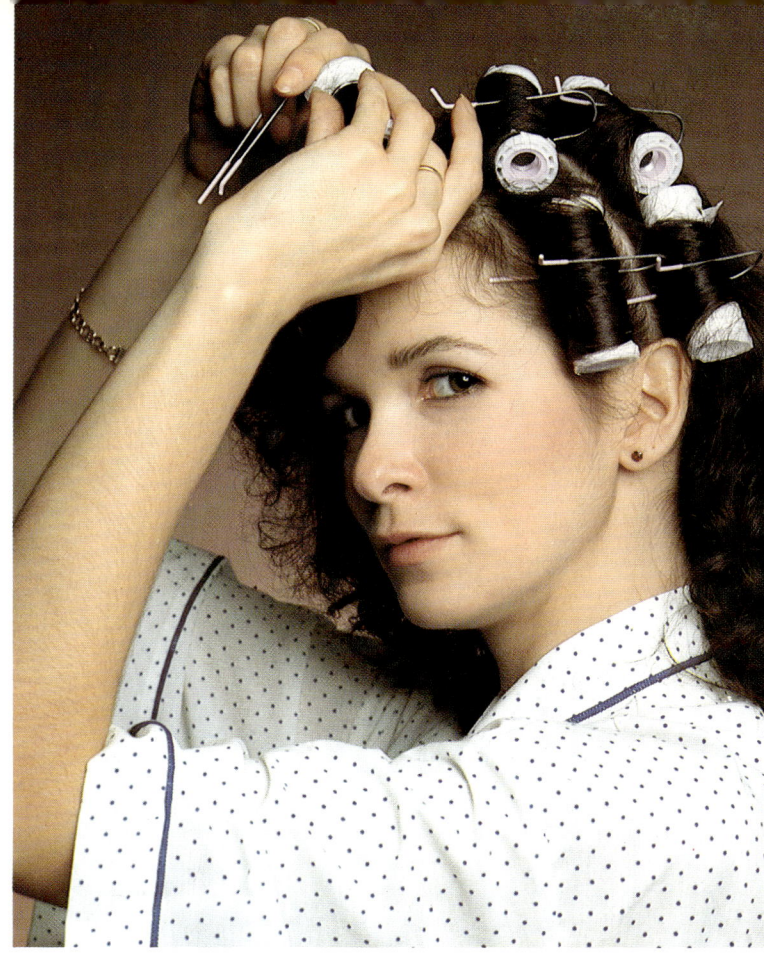
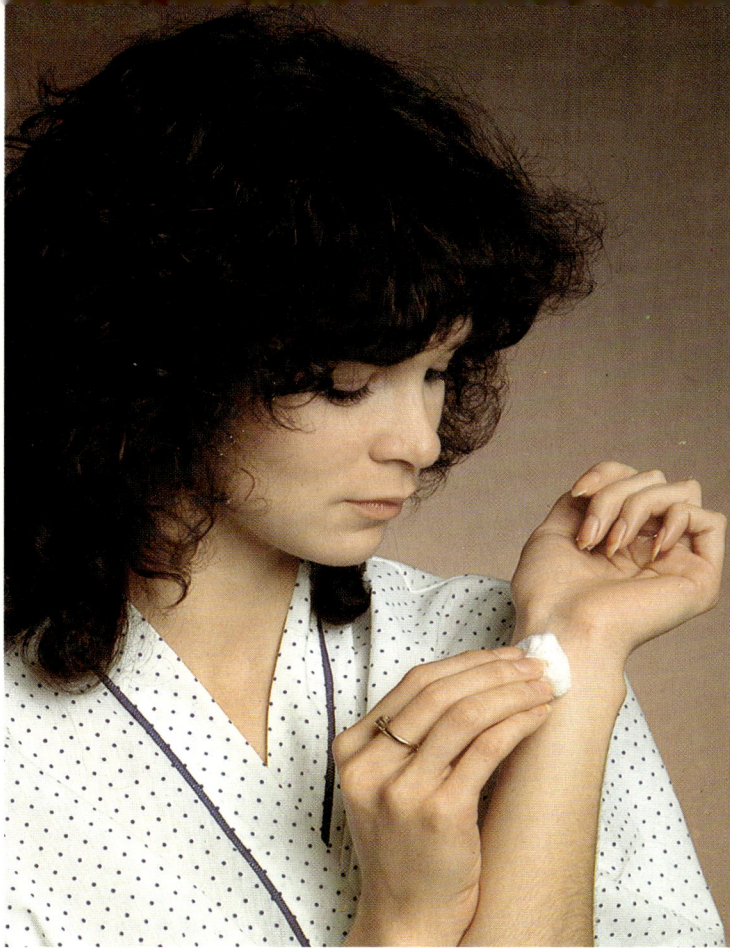

make the effort, do try to keep your hair clean and in good condition. It will help to boost your morale. Pregnancy may have had the effect of making your hair greasy, and the only remedy for this is more frequent washing. Dry shampoo is generally recommended as a means of reviving hair between washes, but this will have a dulling rather than a cleansing effect, and can cause clogging of the hair follicles. If your hair has become drier, be sparing with the shampoo (one application should be enough) and use a conditioner or cream rinse after every wash to prevent it becoming too brittle. As a special treatment, rub olive oil into your hair and wrap your head in hot towels for twenty minutes before washing (put the shampoo straight on to your hair without wetting, or you'll never get the oil out again). Remember that the sun has a drying effect on the hair so wear a scarf or hat for protection if you are sitting out in hot weather.

Temporary tints, mild bleaches, medicated shampoos, setting lotions and hairsprays are all perfectly safe to use during pregnancy in the normal way. It is a good idea to do a patch test on your skin with tints and bleaches, just to make sure you aren't allergic to them. If you do decide you want to use anything more permanent in the way of dyes and bleaches, it is probably better to have this done professionally.

When blow-drying or setting your hair at home, make sure you are sitting comfortably – never stand, as you will inevitably find you are leaning and hunching your shoulders forward, which is both uncomfortable and bad for your posture. Relax at a table with adequate lighting over the mirror and sit on a straight-backed chair so that you don't slump or let your back sag while you are wielding the dryer. Choose a soft, round, pure-bristle brush and try not to over-dry the hair with too much heat from dryers, heated tongs or rollers. If you use heated rollers, make sure that the hair is not wound too tightly round them as they may scratch the surface of the scalp and cause dry hair to break at the roots.

Infections of the scalp

If you find that your scalp itches and flakes badly or you are unfortunate enough to catch lice, never use harsh chemicals (such as parasiticides) without proper advice from a doctor, dermatologist or qualified trichologist. Some of these chemicals could be harmful to the baby should you absorb them by accident into the bloodstream.

A tissue wrapped round each heated roller is a useful tip to protect your hair and scalp. Before using a tint or bleach, do your own patch test to make sure it doesn't cause an allergic reaction.

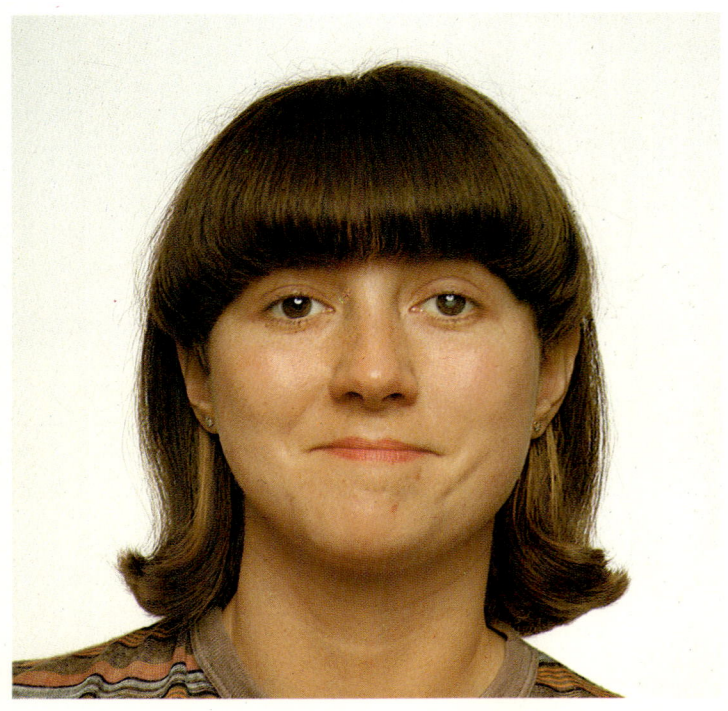

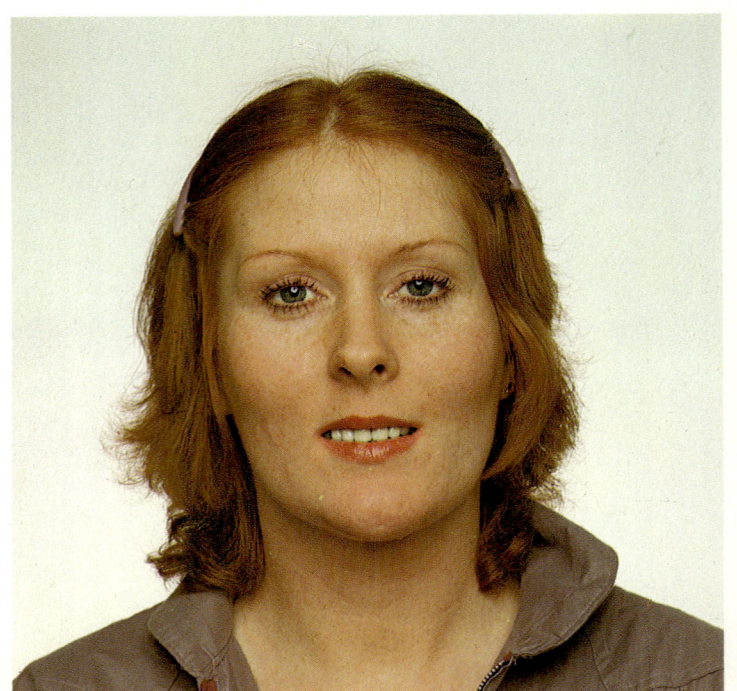

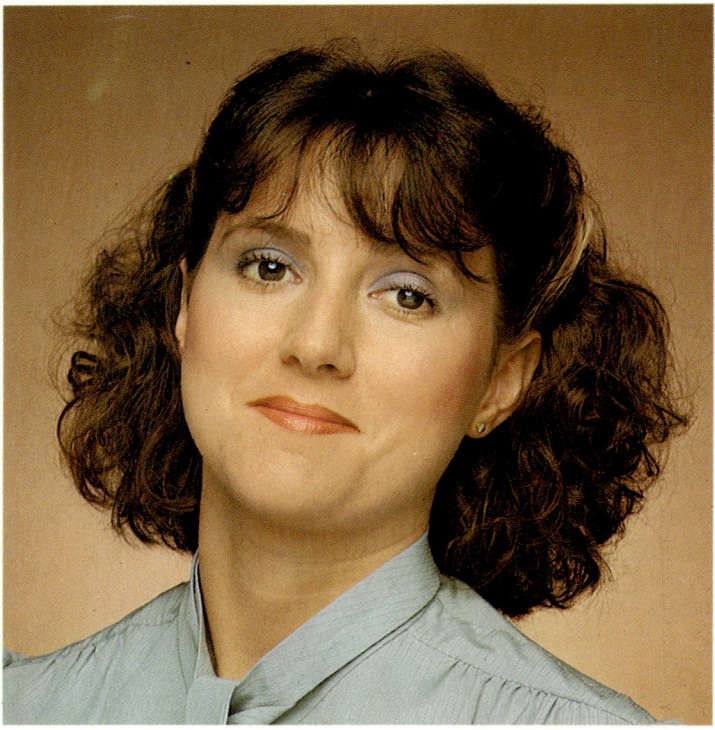

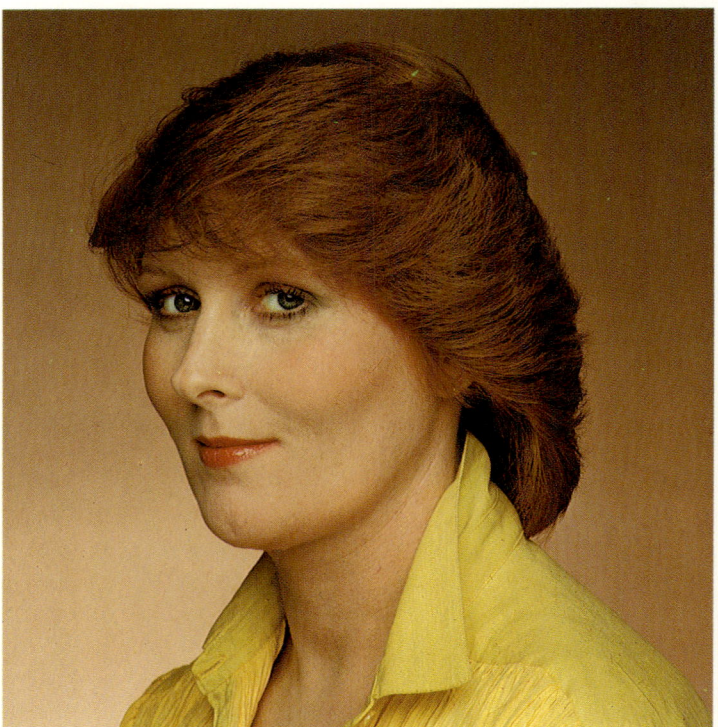

A naturally round face may look even rounder during pregnancy due to the puffiness caused by fluid retention. If this is the case, it is a good idea to avoid a heavy straight style, which will tend to emphasize plump cheeks and a slightly double chin. The style we show aims at a softer look, and by brushing the hair up at the sides and making it much fuller at the back, emphasis is drawn away from the face, which has a slimming effect. These casual waves are achieved by finger drying the hair – or by a light perm if your hair is dead straight.

Very fine hair is always a bit of a problem to look after, but could be more so now if it becomes lank and oily. A layered style will help to give it a thicker texture (hair all the same length tends to lie flat to the head) and blow drying using a small round brush provides more body. This style with the hair swept gently backwards is simple but attractive and is an easy one to do yourself at home.

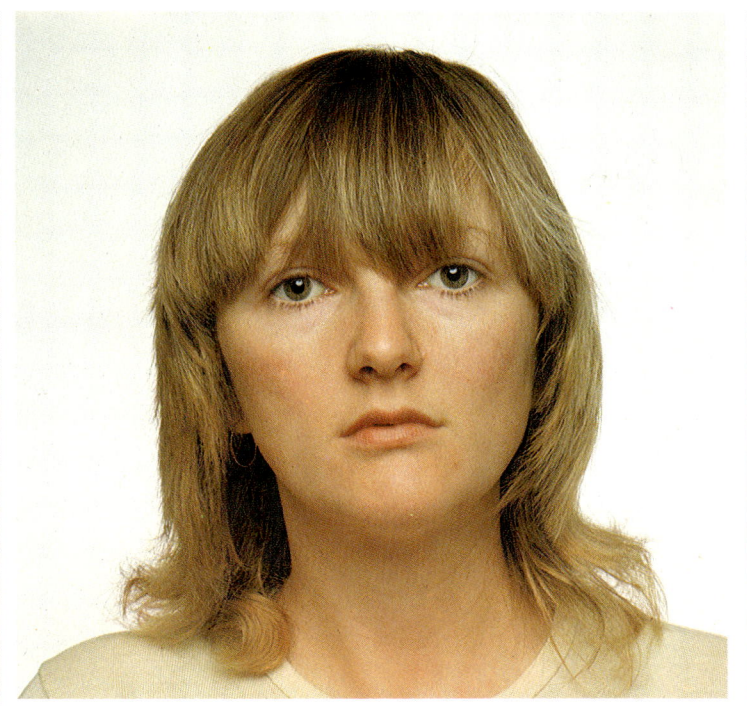

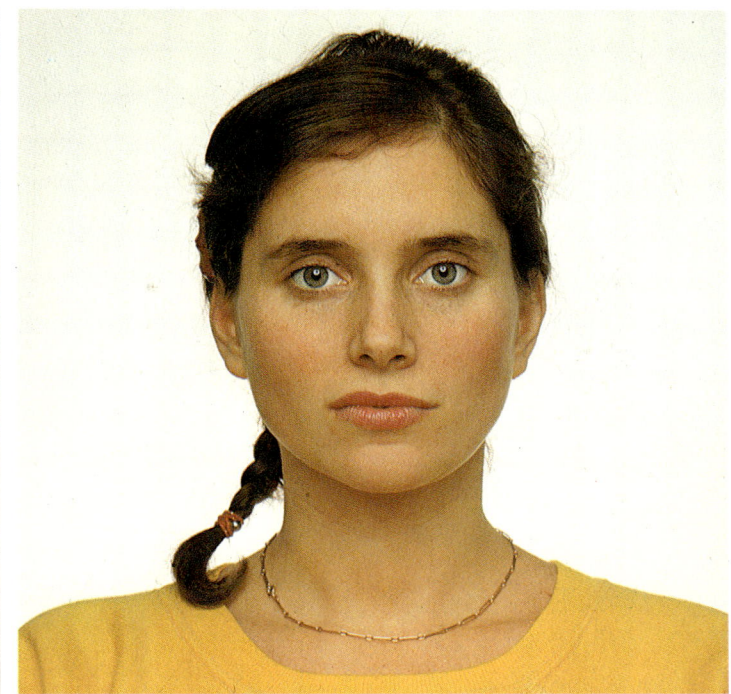

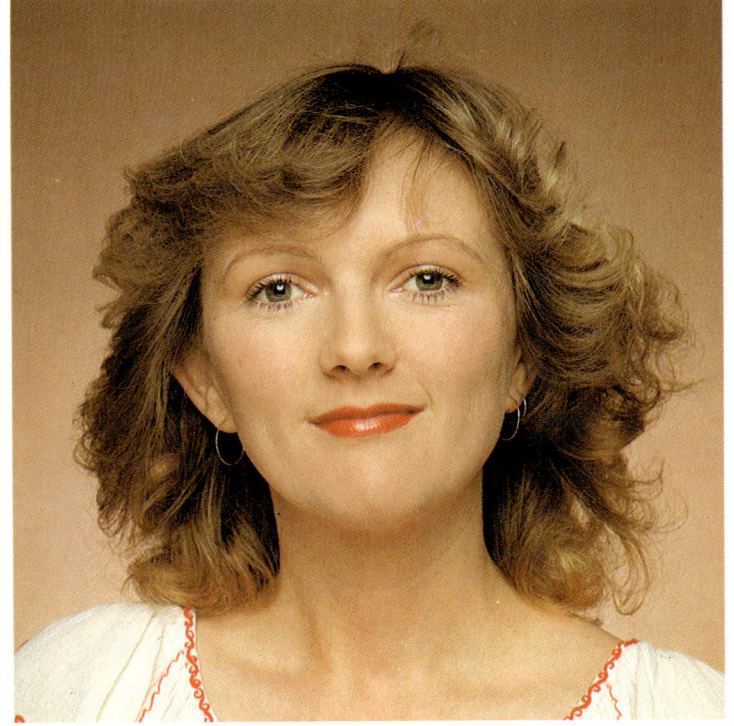

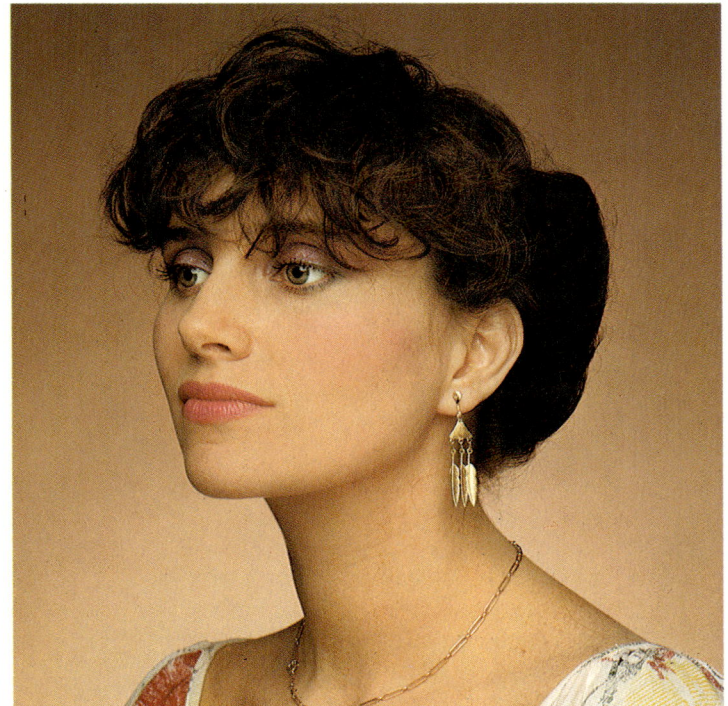

If you've always yearned for flowing waves or bouncing curls, this could be the time to cast caution to the winds and try them, because a fuller hairstyle will flatter your face and make you appear less bottom heavy! If your hair is not naturally curly, a light perm is ideal so that you can finger dry your hair when you wash it yourself – no rollers required. But if you are unsure if this sort of style will suit you, ask your hairdresser to curl your hair naturally first, before embarking on a perm.

A glamorous look is always a boost and this elegant evening style is not difficult to achieve. Divide your hair into five sections – one at the front, one at each side, and two at the back. Put the front hair into small heated rollers (if not already curly) and backcomb each of the other sections at the roots, lightly spraying them with hairspray. Fold over the back sections to make a roll and grip firmly, then sweep the side sections back over the roll, tucking in the ends and pinning them so that no joins are visible. Gently brush out the front hair to curl naturally over your forehead.

Fashion

Being pregnant doesn't mean you have to look frumpy, dowdy or unfashionable. Nor does it necessarily mean you have to change your normal style of dress. True, the popular image of a pregnant woman is one who is dressed in an all-enveloping smock and many people do like this kind of comfortable, easy style. But if you have always been a jeans-and-sweater girl there is no reason to be different now.

Adapting your wardrobe for the first months

Unfortunately there is just no way of foretelling exactly how large you are eventually going to be, nor when you are actually going to be 'showing' your pregnancy. Some women look pregnant at three to four months, whereas others go unnoticed well into their sixth month. The most obvious change is of course your tummy, but quite early on you will probably find that your waistline thickens and your breasts become larger. In fact, it is those first few months that are the most awkward. You know that you're pregnant and will feel larger than you look to others. Waistbands will be tight and blouses uncomfortable across the bust. Wearing tight clothes won't harm your baby, the discomfort will merely make you feel bigger than you are. So don't go on struggling into tight jeans, straight skirts and slinky dresses. But before you dash out and panic buy expensive maternity clothes, take stock of your wardrobe. Have a good look at everything and see what can be altered, adapted or used as it is.

For casual wear at home, jeans can be adapted for a while by clipping a pair of men's braces to the front and back and leaving the zip undone, with a loose, undarted shirt or baggy T-shirt or jumper to hide the gap. If you want to wear trousers throughout pregnancy you can convert them by letting out the darts, taking off the waistband and zip, and inserting bands of wide, soft elastic ribbing in the front, back and side seams.

You can go on wearing boiler suits and dungarees during much of your pregnancy and towelling track suits in primary colours are fun and comfortable. If the elastic at the

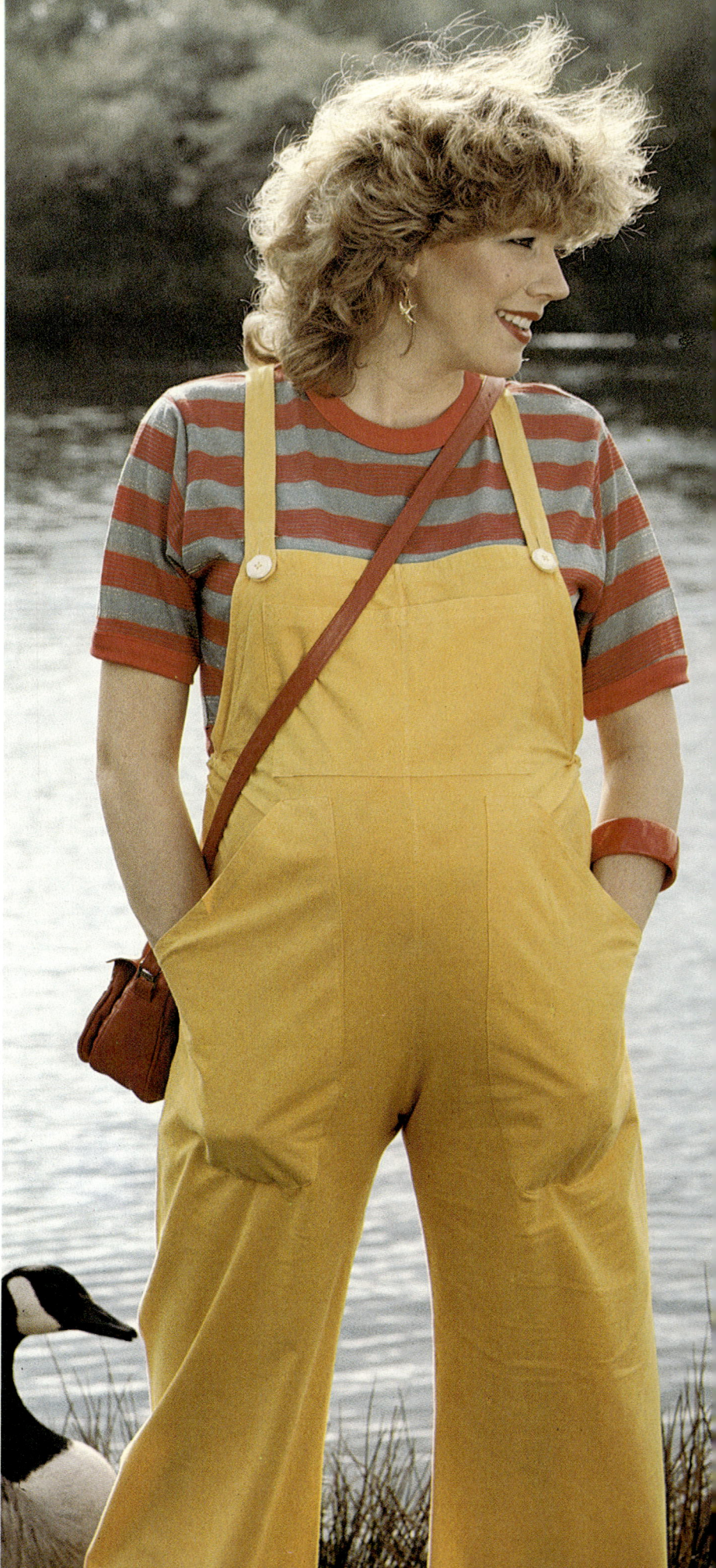

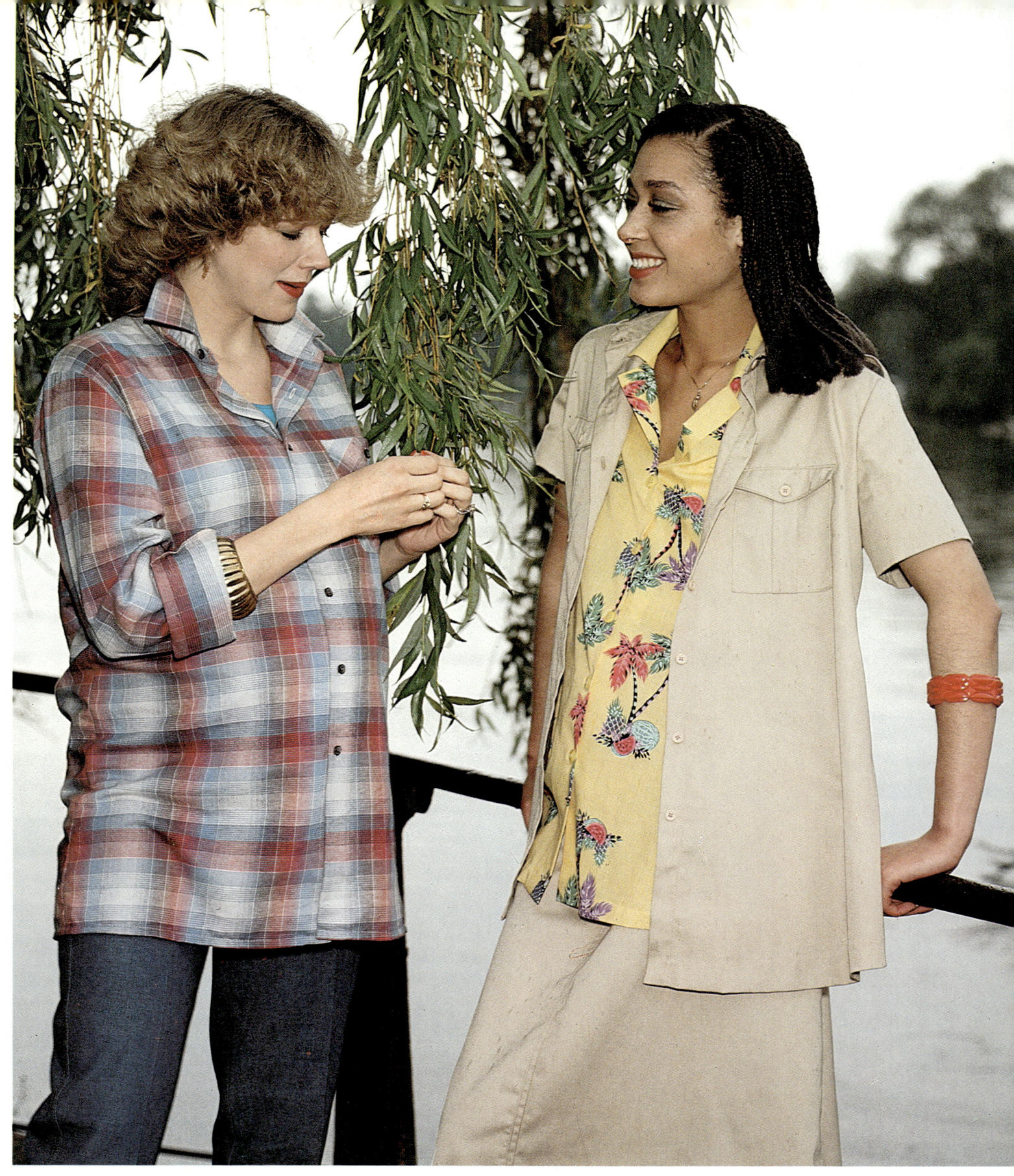

Casual

Dungarees allow plenty of room for expansion and the colours can be as cheerful as you like. If smocks aren't your style then you might invest in maternity jeans or skirts (which have a soft elastic panel at the front) with a smart selection of extra-large shirts to cover the bulge.

Day wear

If you can't find a maternity dress that suits you, don't despair – none of the clothes on this page were designed for expectant mothers. Look out for undarted shifts, loose dresses pleated or gathered at the shoulder, and for A-line macs and jackets.

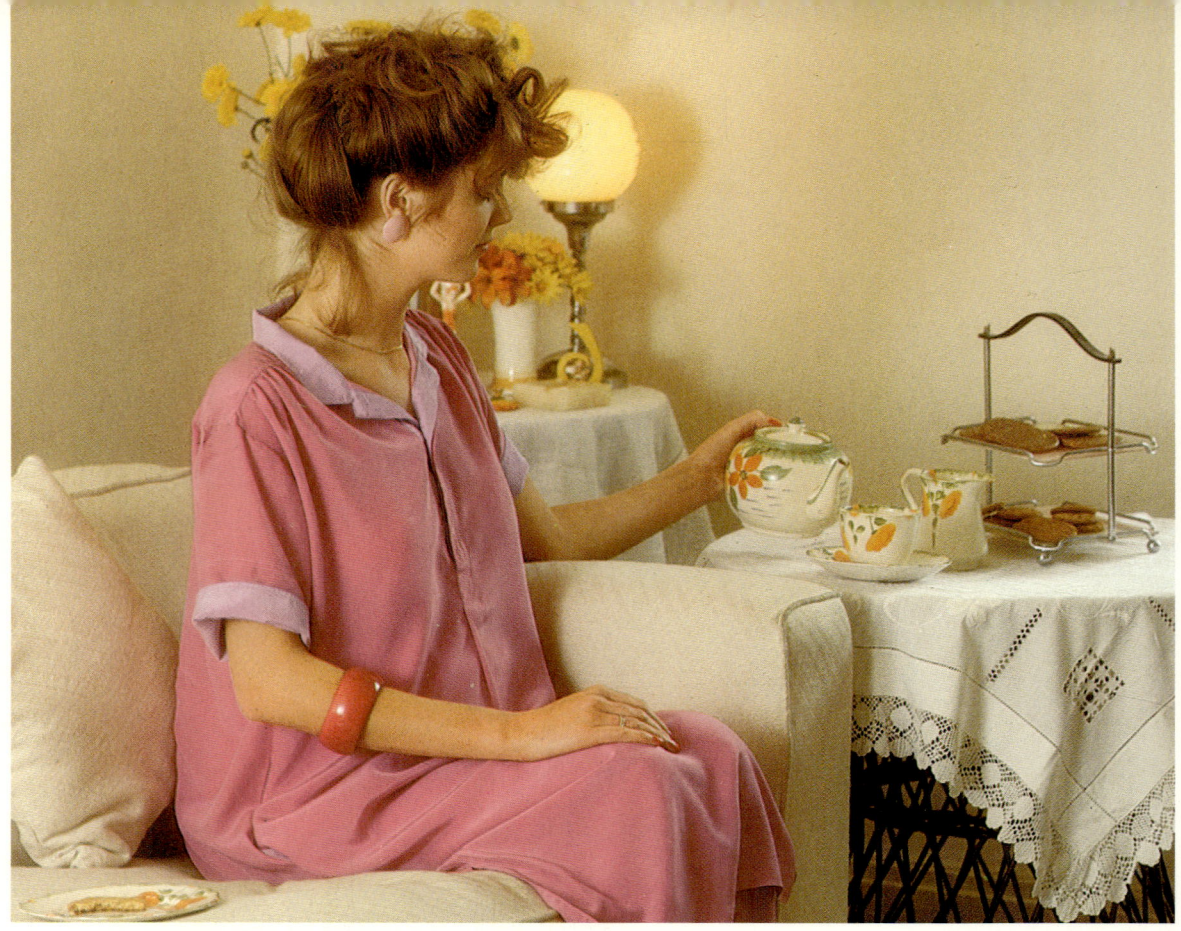

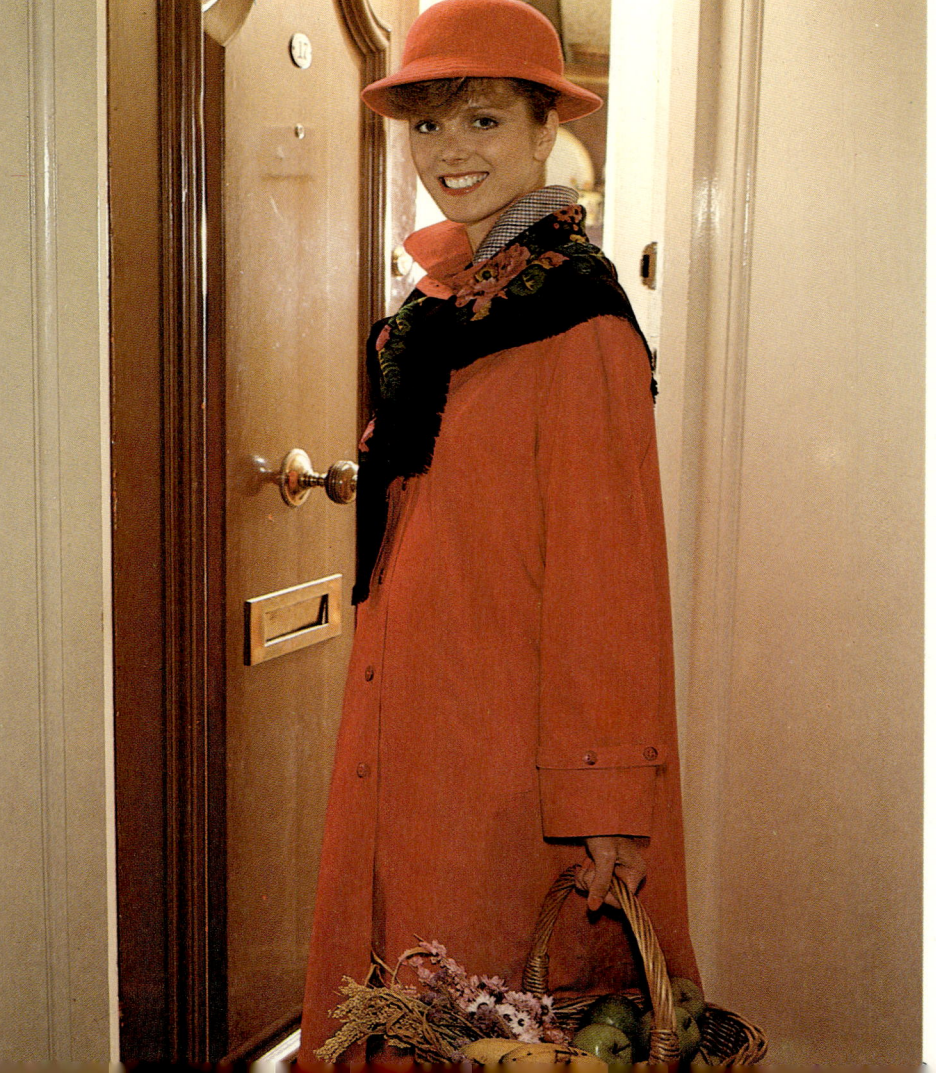

waist feels too tight, replace it with drawstrings. Wrap-around skirts are useful for the early months and many loose dresses with undarted busts can be worn without belts – or cut down to make baggy tops. When your tummy is only just noticeable, sweater and shirt dresses look elegant with the material 'bloused' up over the belt, which can be worn 1920s-style low down on your hips.

Maternity and non-maternity clothes

When you start to look for new clothes you may find that there isn't a great deal of choice – and what there is could be expensive. However maternity styles are improving and if you hunt around you should be able to come up with one or two attractive clothes, whether dresses, suits, trouser suits or even maternity culottes.

If you like to wear jeans, maternity trousers are now becoming more fashionably cut, look for a good quality pair with a large elastic panel in the front and plenty of give at the back. They may be expensive – the best-looking ones are usually French or American – but you can wear them virtually every day throughout

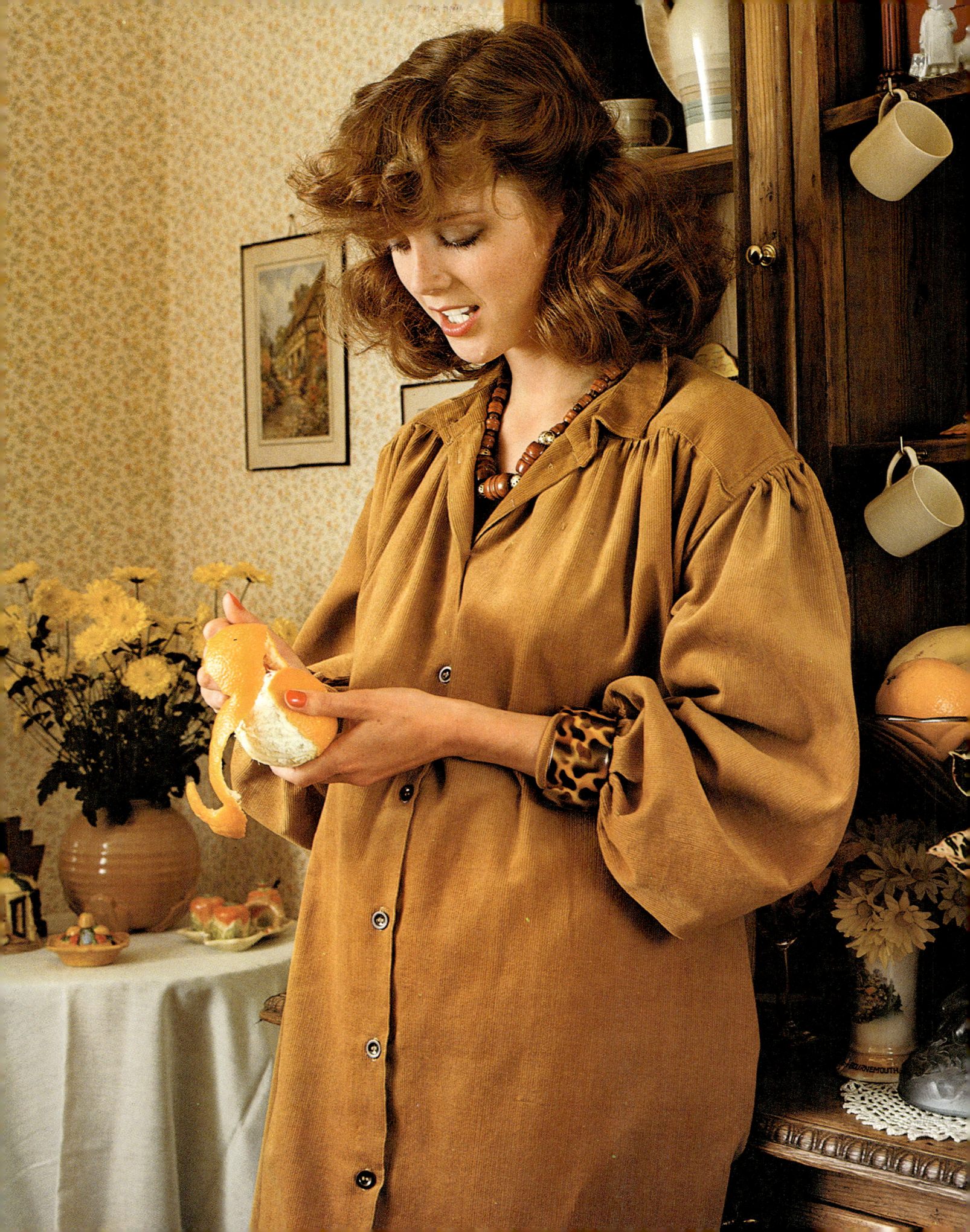

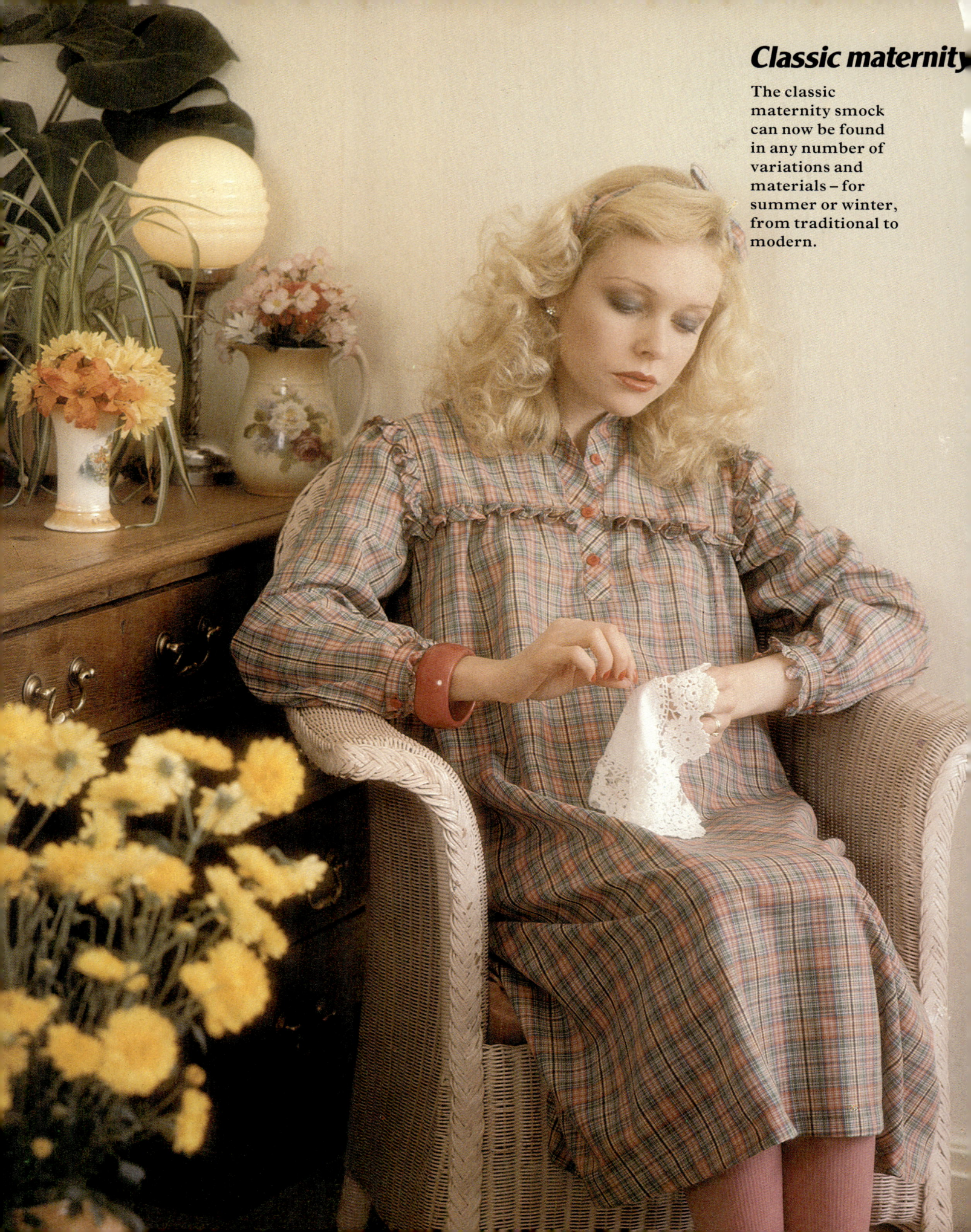

Classic maternity

The classic maternity smock can now be found in any number of variations and materials – for summer or winter, from traditional to modern.

the second half of your pregnancy with a variety of different tops and T-shirts.

If you can't find what you want among the maternity clothes, look out for dresses that are pin-tucked or pleated from the shoulders, or, in the summer, loose sun dresses with a shirred elastic yoke over the bust. Pinafore dresses are very versatile worn with jumpers or shirts in the day and silky blouses in the evening. You can also find dresses in soft, Indian cotton or cheesecloth, which are loose and flowing, or an elegant kaftan which, pregnant or not, will make a useful addition to your wardrobe.

Wear bright, cheerful colours if you are happy in them. But remember that large prints and stripes will tend to make you look bigger. If you prefer a more subtle, feminine look, choose soft, muted prints in small flowery patterns. Black and navy blue always look smart but avoid dark browns and greys which can be drab.

Fabrics should be easy to wash and not too thick, since your higher metabolic rate and increased blood circulation will probably make you feel warmer than usual, even in the winter. If natural fibres are too expensive, choose blends such as cotton-polyester or wool-acrylic rather than pure synthetics – and nothing too clingy!

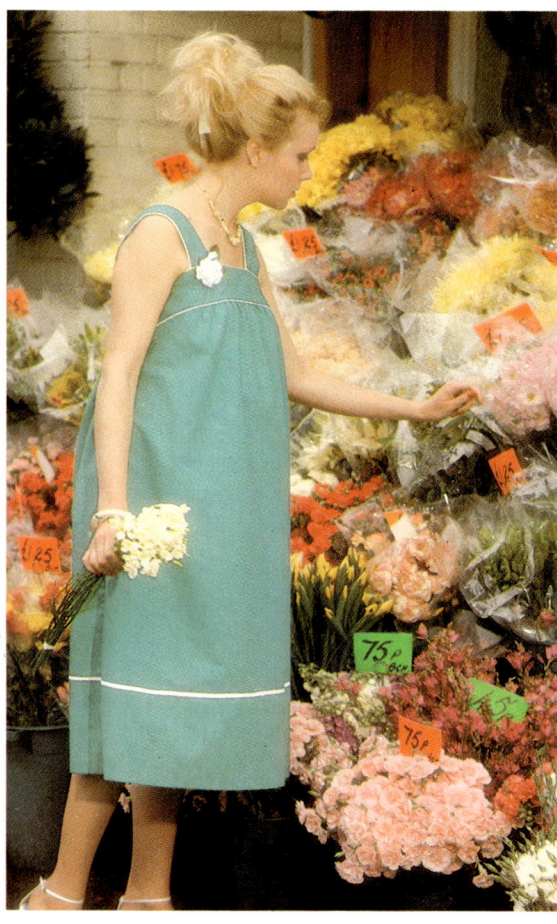

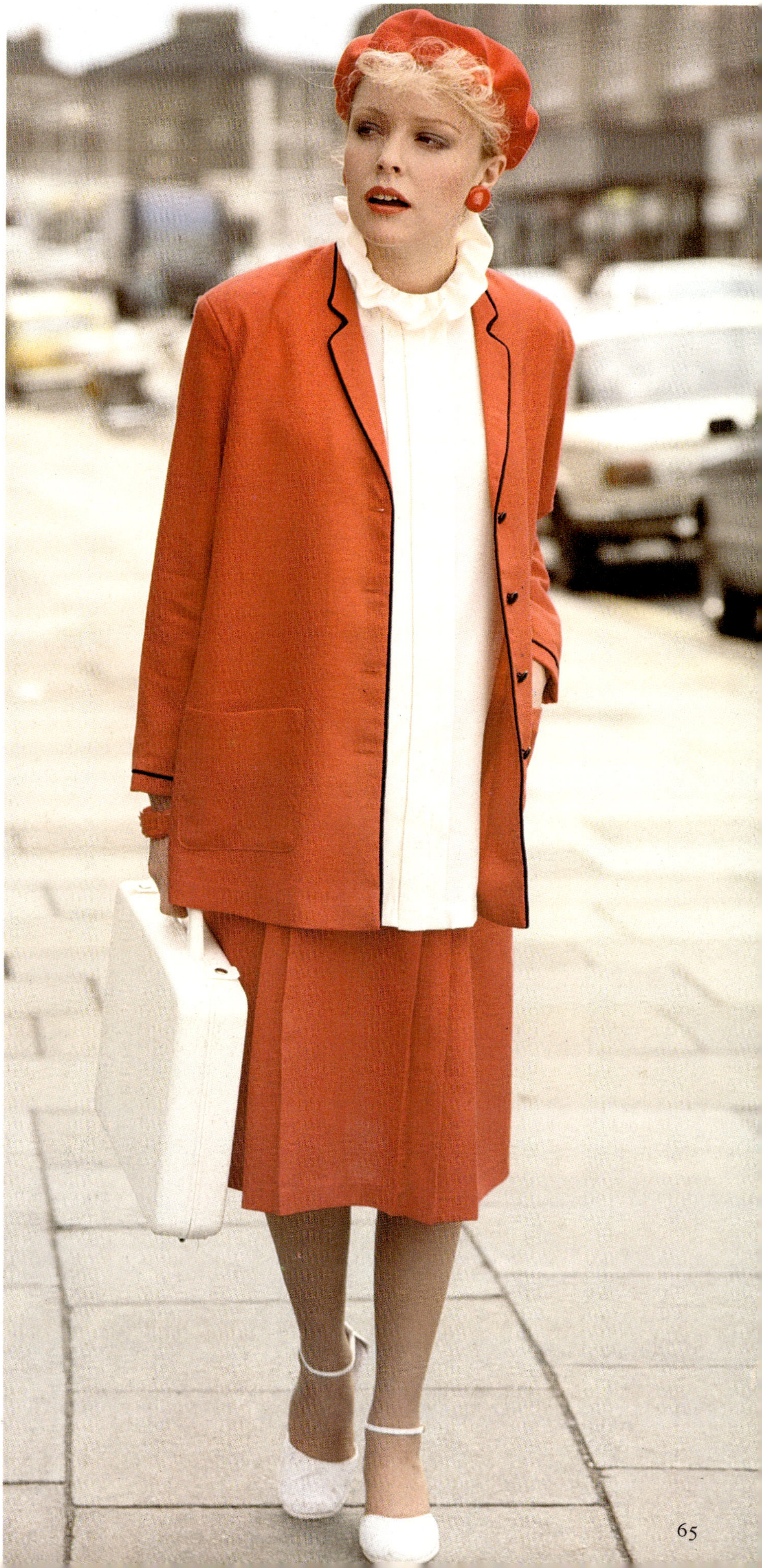

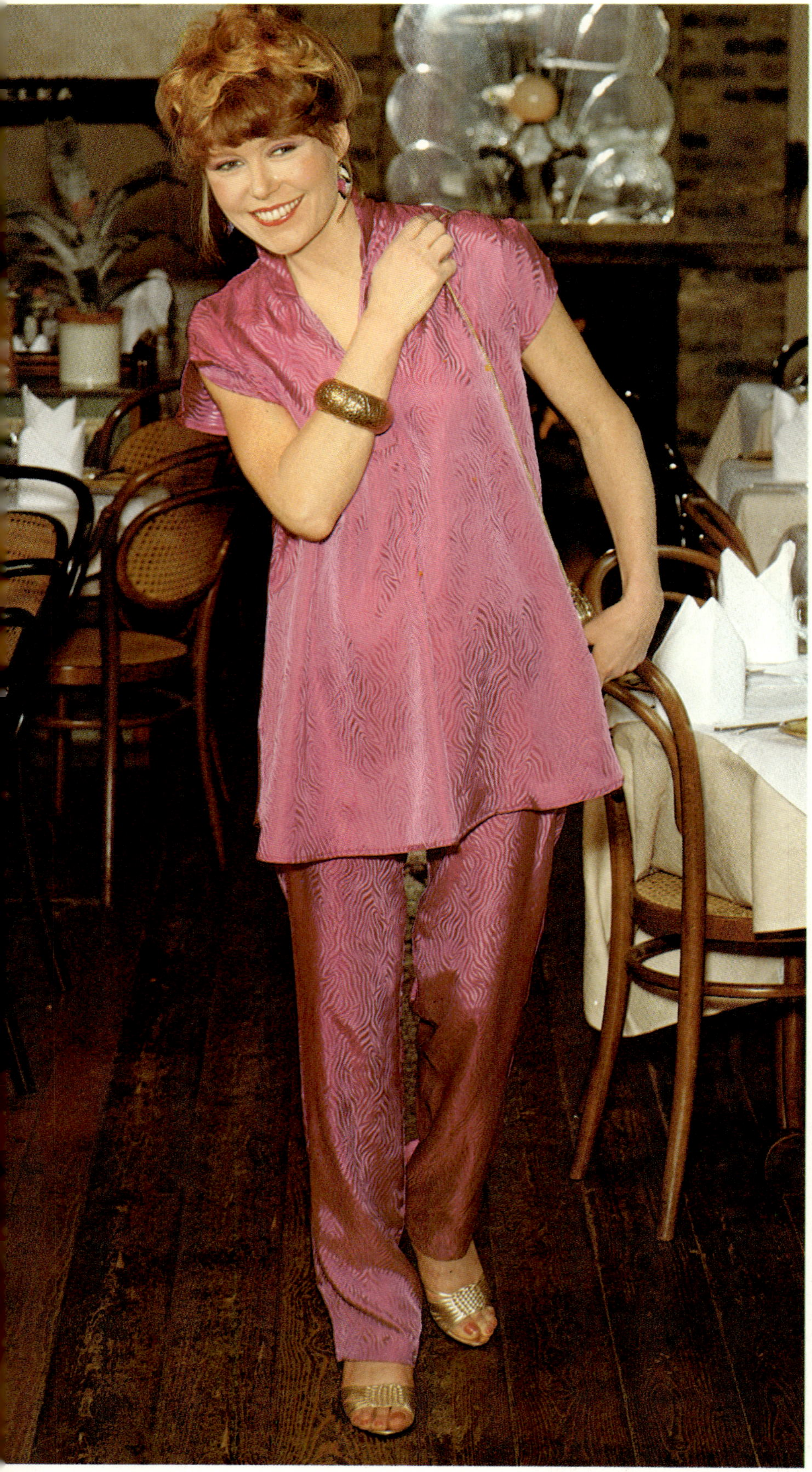

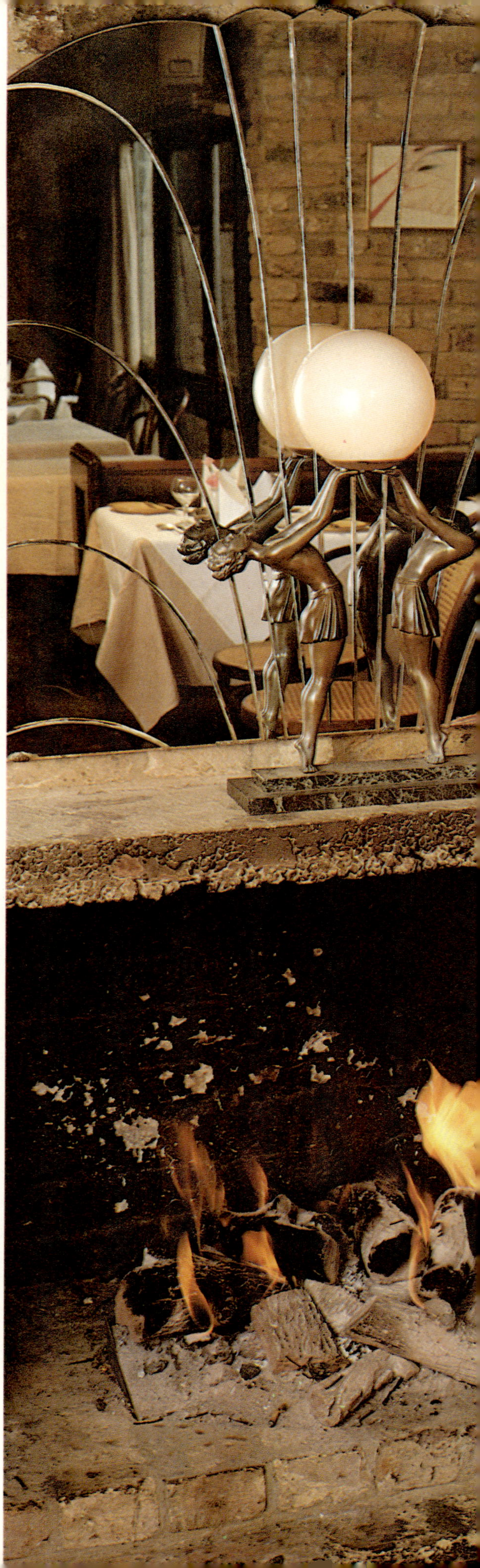

Evening

For a special
evening occasion

you can afford to be
a little more daring
with colours,
patterns or styles.

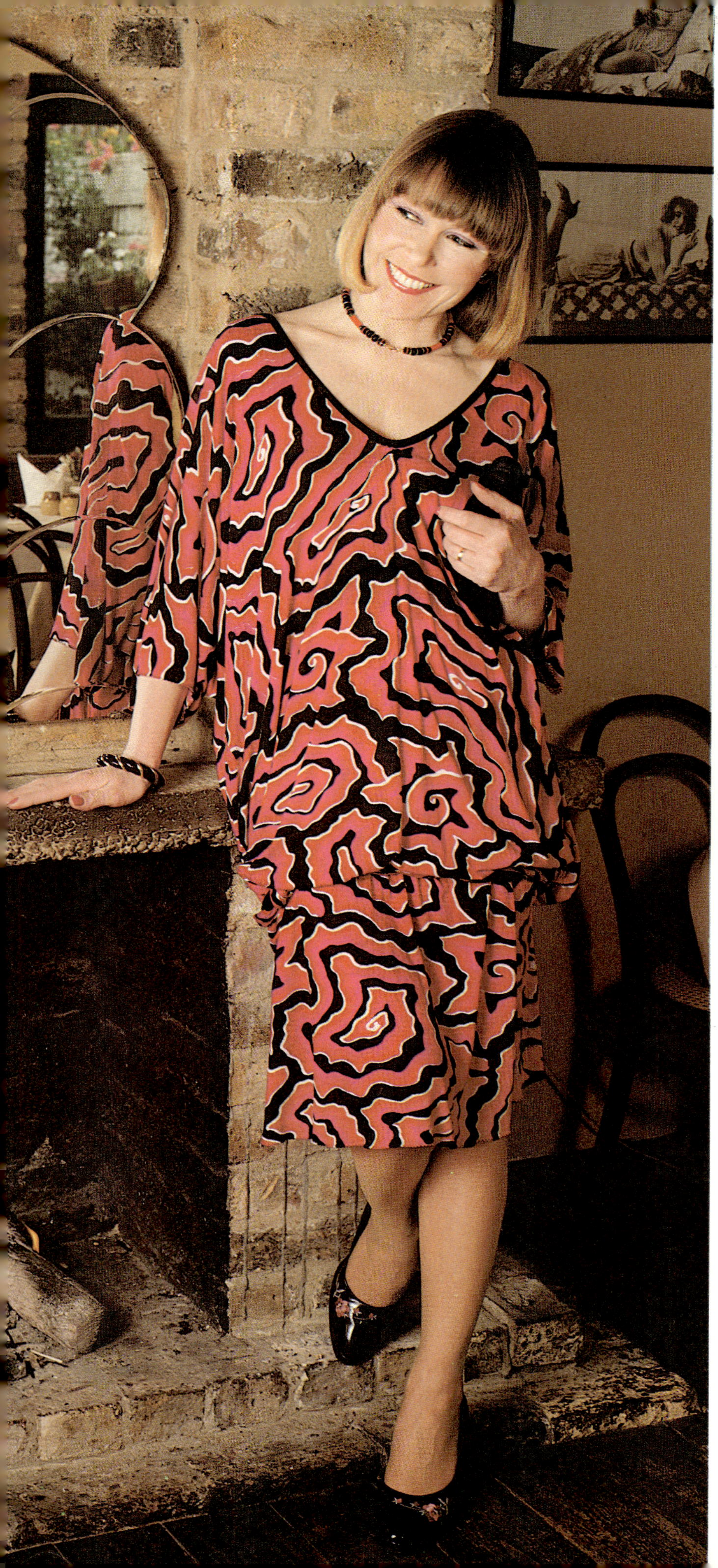

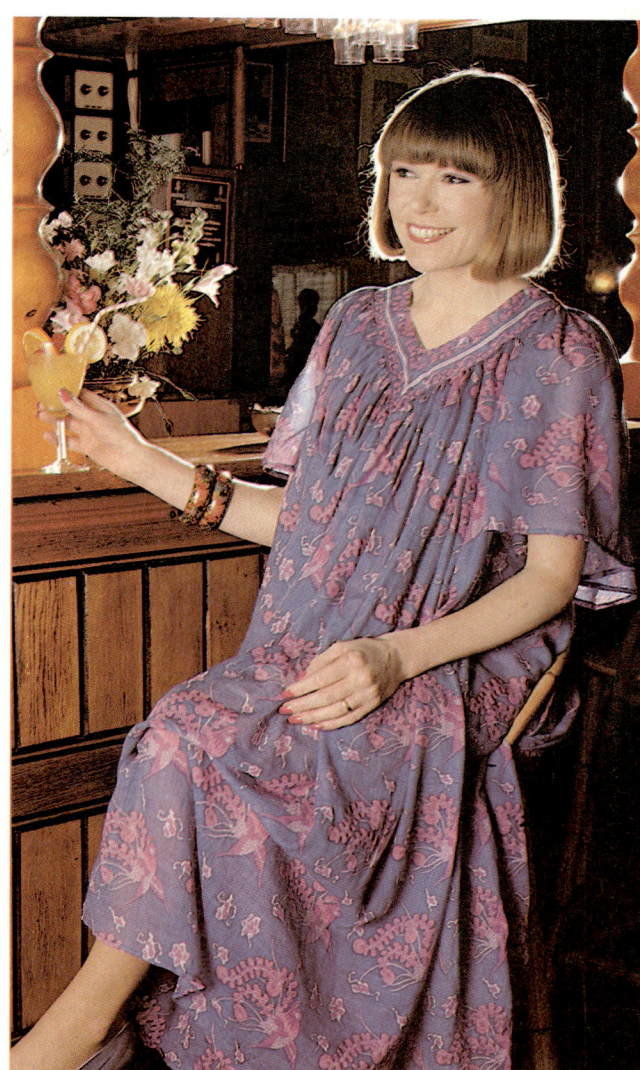

Evening wear

Kaftans, which have already been mentioned, can be dressed up or down to suit most occasions. On the other hand, now may be the moment to make the most of an unaccustomed cleavage, so if you need a new evening dress why not boost your morale with a low-cut, glamorous dress in a silky washable fabric. There are quite a few styles that can be gathered in with a belt and so worn afterwards when you have regained your waistline.

Coats and jackets

You probably won't want to invest in a new winter coat while you are pregnant, but unwaisted swing-shape or A-line raincoats, capes and hip-length loose or blouson jackets are all useful and concealing – as are unwaisted fur coats if you are lucky enough to have one in your wardrobe!

On the beach

There are pretty maternity swimsuits on the market to conceal your tummy, but if you are happy to show it off, there is no reason why you shouldn't wear an ordinary bikini. The sight of a bare, pregnant stomach on the beach upsets very few people, so you don't have to pass up the opportunity of getting a nice brown body. If you are self-conscious though, a large T-shirt knotted at the side, a kanga, or strapless sun-top will cover you up and look attractive.

Underclothes and nightwear

We've already talked about bras and other support garments in an earlier chapter (see pages 24–9) so this section deals with 'fashion' underwear. Pants are most comfortable worn below the tummy, so stretchy bikini briefs are best. Buy cotton rather than synthetics as you are less likely to sweat in them. Tights can be worn throughout pregnancy so long as you find them comfortable; they should have a lot of 'give' so that you can pull the gusset right up under your bust. Stockings tend to become impractical as you grow larger, simply because the suspender belt will feel tight and ungainly. You should never wear garters to keep your stockings up; this will constrict the blood flow in your legs and could cause varicose veins. If you like to wear socks with trousers, make sure the elastic isn't too tight and keep them loosely rolled down if necessary – or better still wear ankle socks in cheerful colours.

Anything loose and airy is suitable for nightwear. If you are not a nightie person, a large T-shirt or ordinary man's shirt with the collar and cuffs removed are comfortable alternatives. But if you are buying with your hospital confinement in mind, two or three nighties or loose-fitting pyjamas with front openings for breastfeeding are essential. Don't be tempted by slinky négligées in synthetic materials as they will make you sweat – hospitals are invariably hot-houses.

Footwear

The combination of your increased weight and the softening of your ligaments during pregnancy means that your feet will need

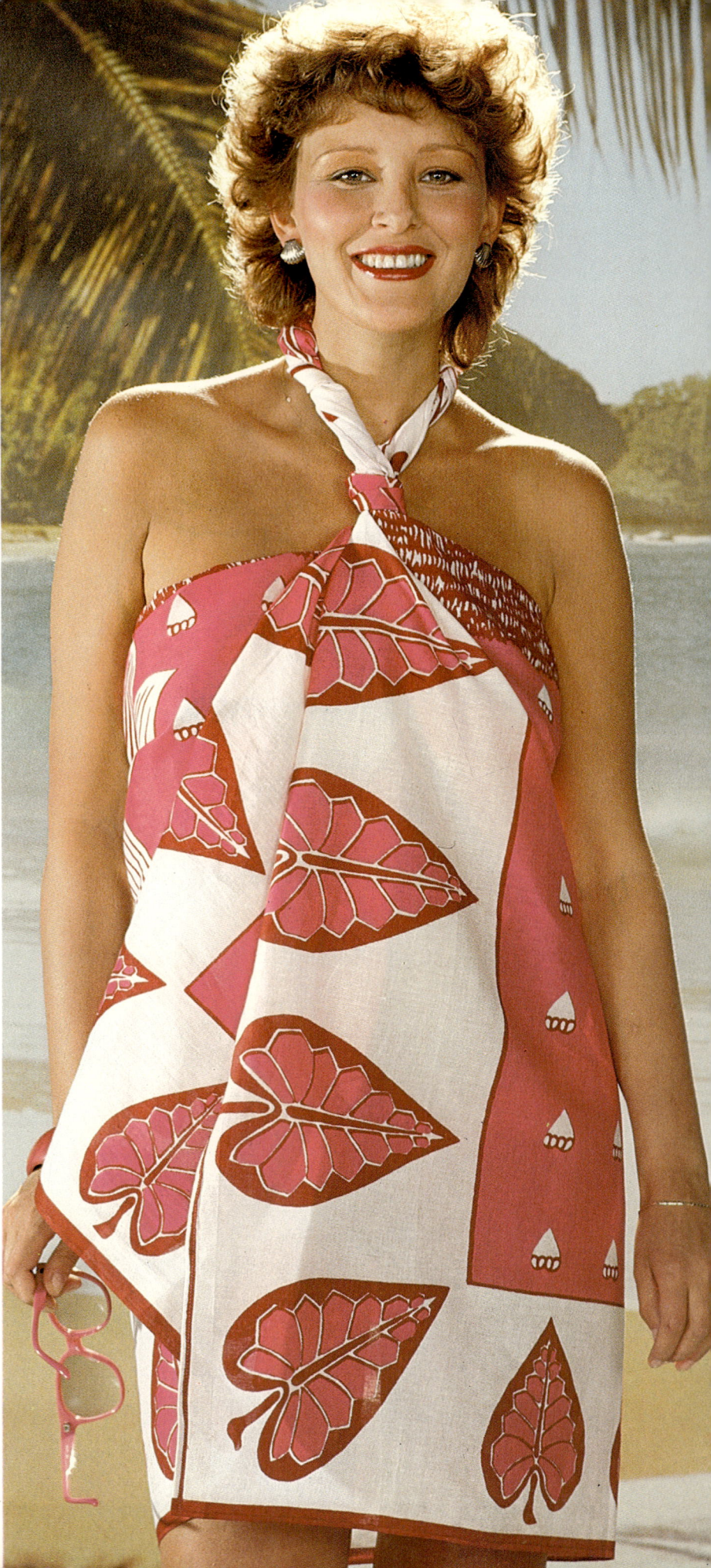

Swimwear

Attractive ideas for beach cover-ups: (left) a kanga – just a huge scarf, (below) an enormous T-shirt knotted at the hip.

extra support and comfort. Buy new shoes half a size larger than usual to allow for expansion. High heels are bad for your feet and could be dangerous since they affect your balance by throwing your weight forward. So choose from the lower-heeled styles, and preferably shoes with straps, laces or some other fastening. Boots should have chunky heels and be supportive yet

wide enough across the instep in case your feet swell. Check that they are not too tight at the ankle or calf. Summer sandals are fine as long as they are comfortable and reasonably supportive. For round the house, wooden exercise sandals, flip flops or no shoes are three quite good ways to exercise your feet, but avoid slippers and mules, they are no benefit at all.

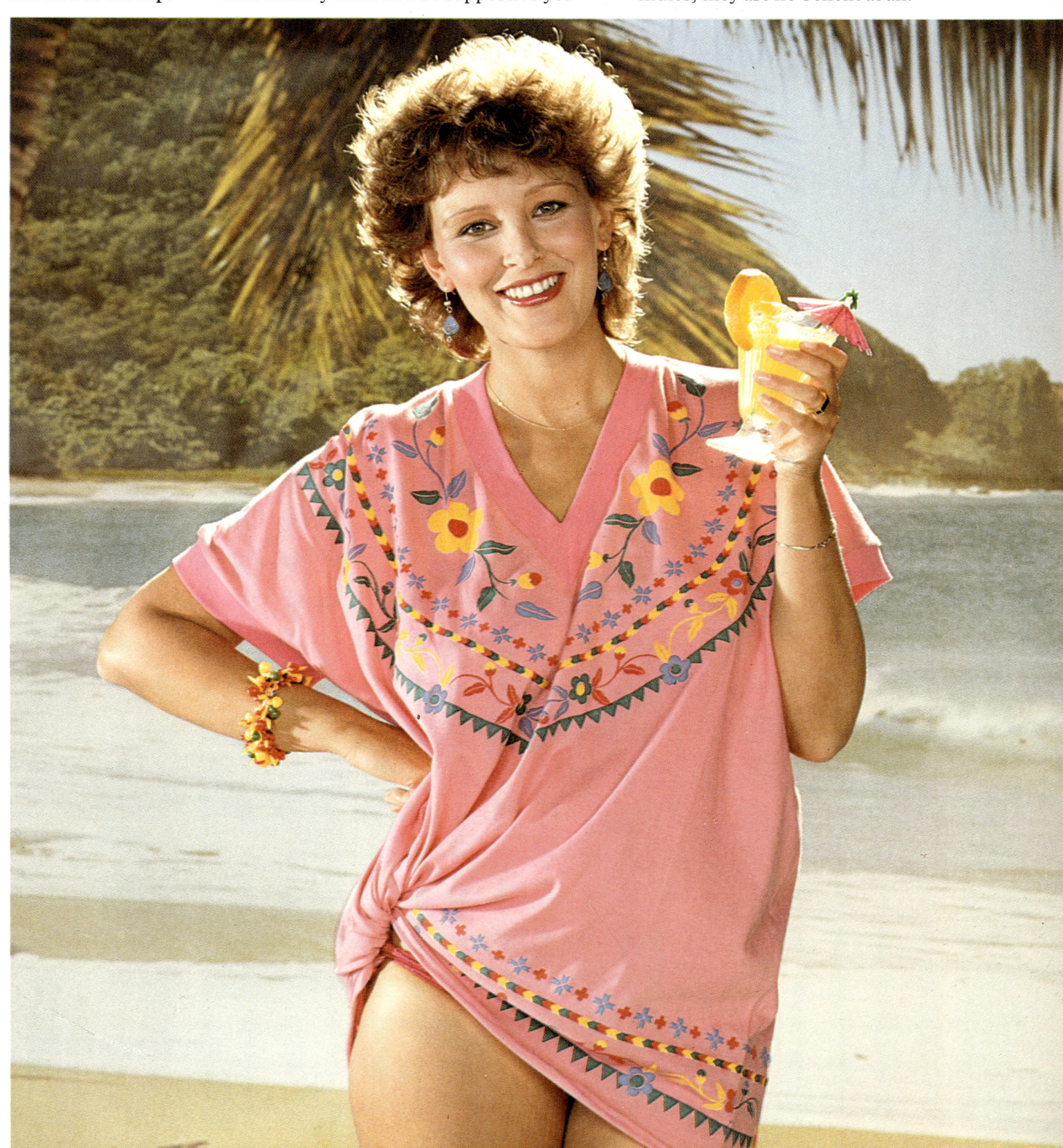

The choice of accessories hardly depends on your shape so you can really go to town here. A pretty straw hat for the summer, berets for the winter, colourful scarves, tights and inexpensive jewellery are all invaluable. Just a pair of brightly coloured socks will cheer an outfit up! Shoes can be fun too, but they must be low-heeled styles that give your feet proper support.

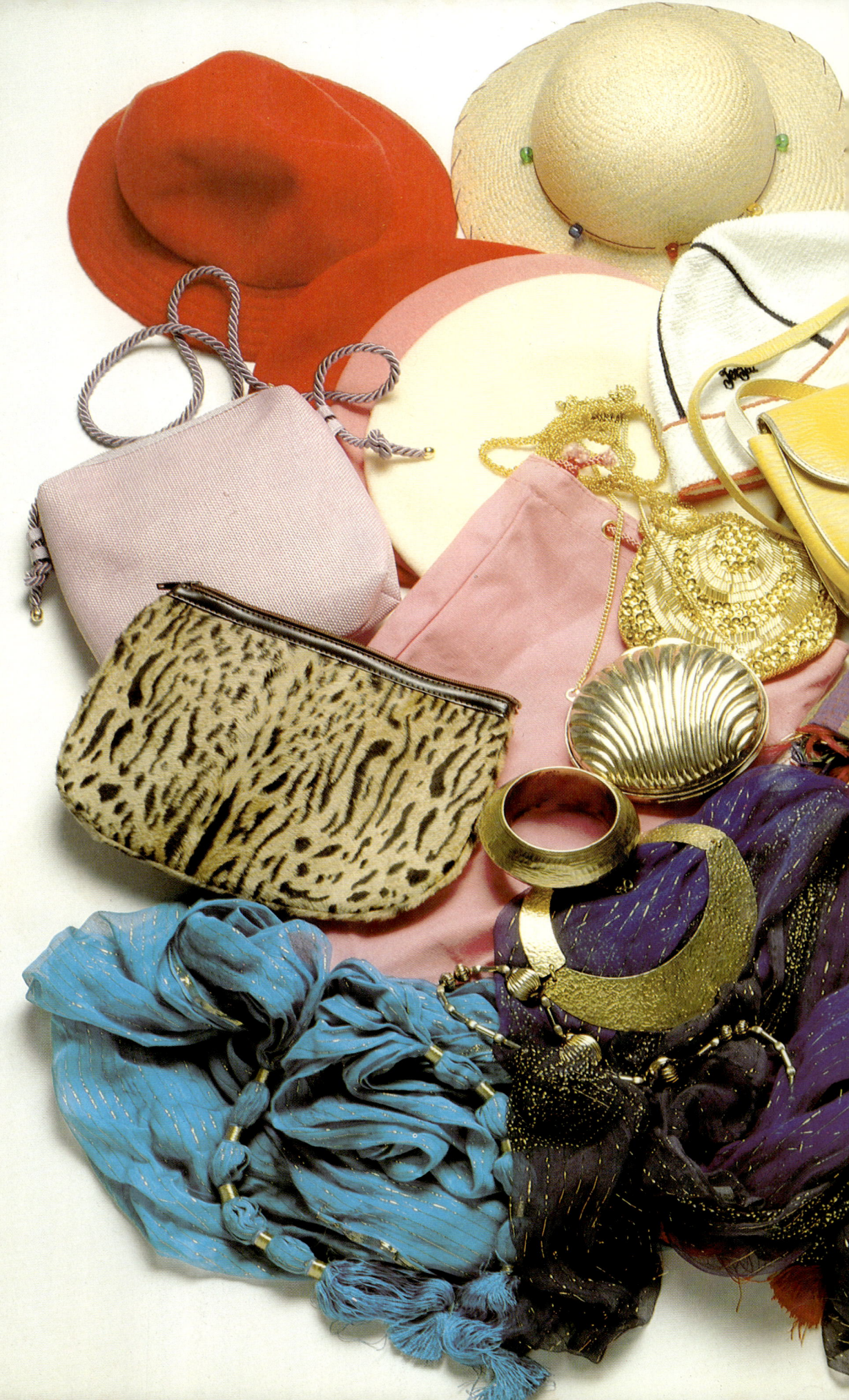

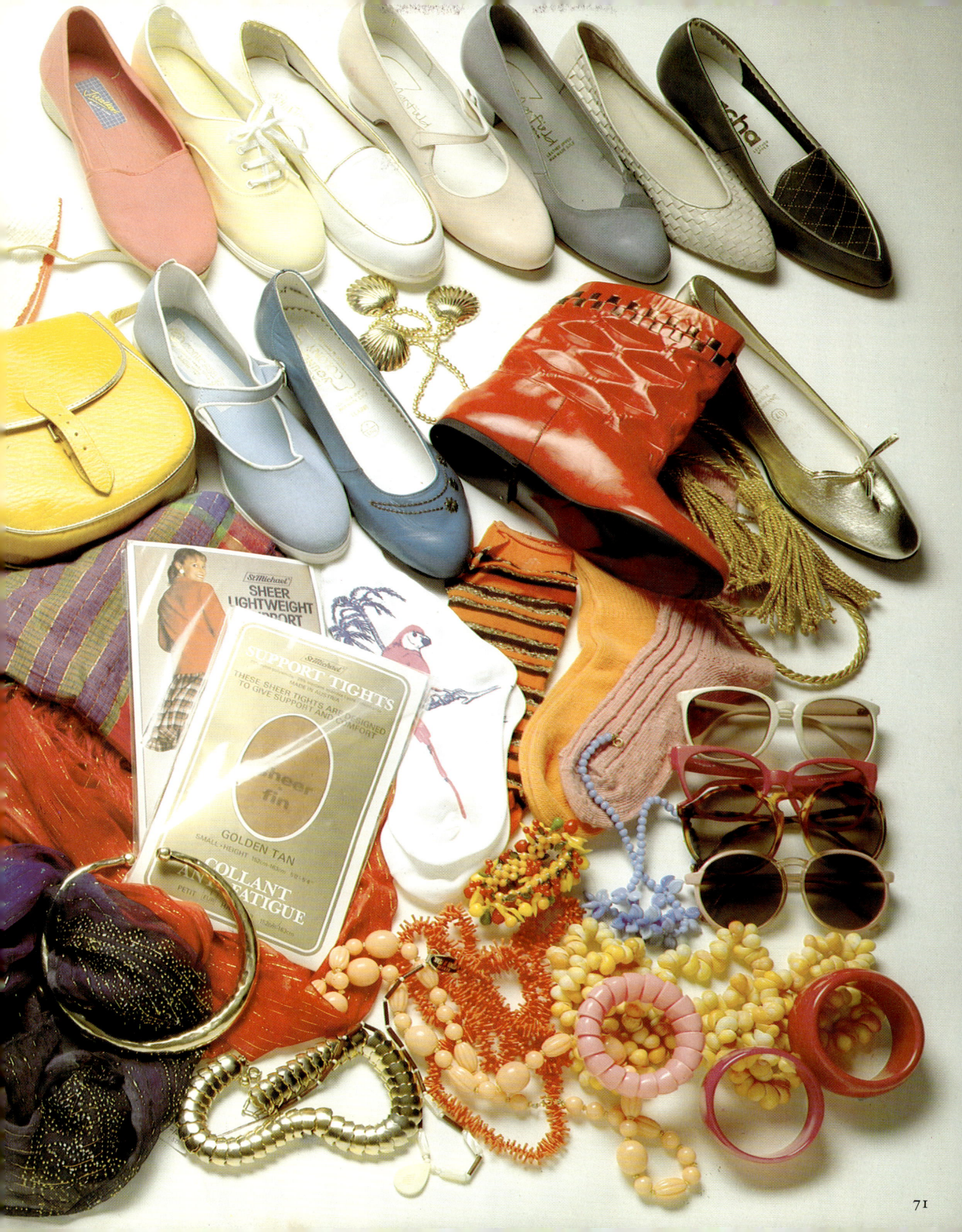

Family and Household

Having a baby requires a certain amount of organization of both home and family to prepare them for the coming event and for your new way of life afterwards. Everyone will want to give you advice about the best way to do things, which can be rather confusing, and sometimes annoying, especially if you have firm ideas of your own about whether you are going to breast or bottle feed, whether or not you are going back to work immediately, and so on. Stick to your guns, but remember that situations concerning those closest to you may arise that need careful handling.

Keeping the family happy

The most important change in attitude to pregnancy over the past few years has been towards the father's role. Up to about fifteen years ago, a husband would duly take his wife to the hospital when the time arrived, but he would not be invited to see

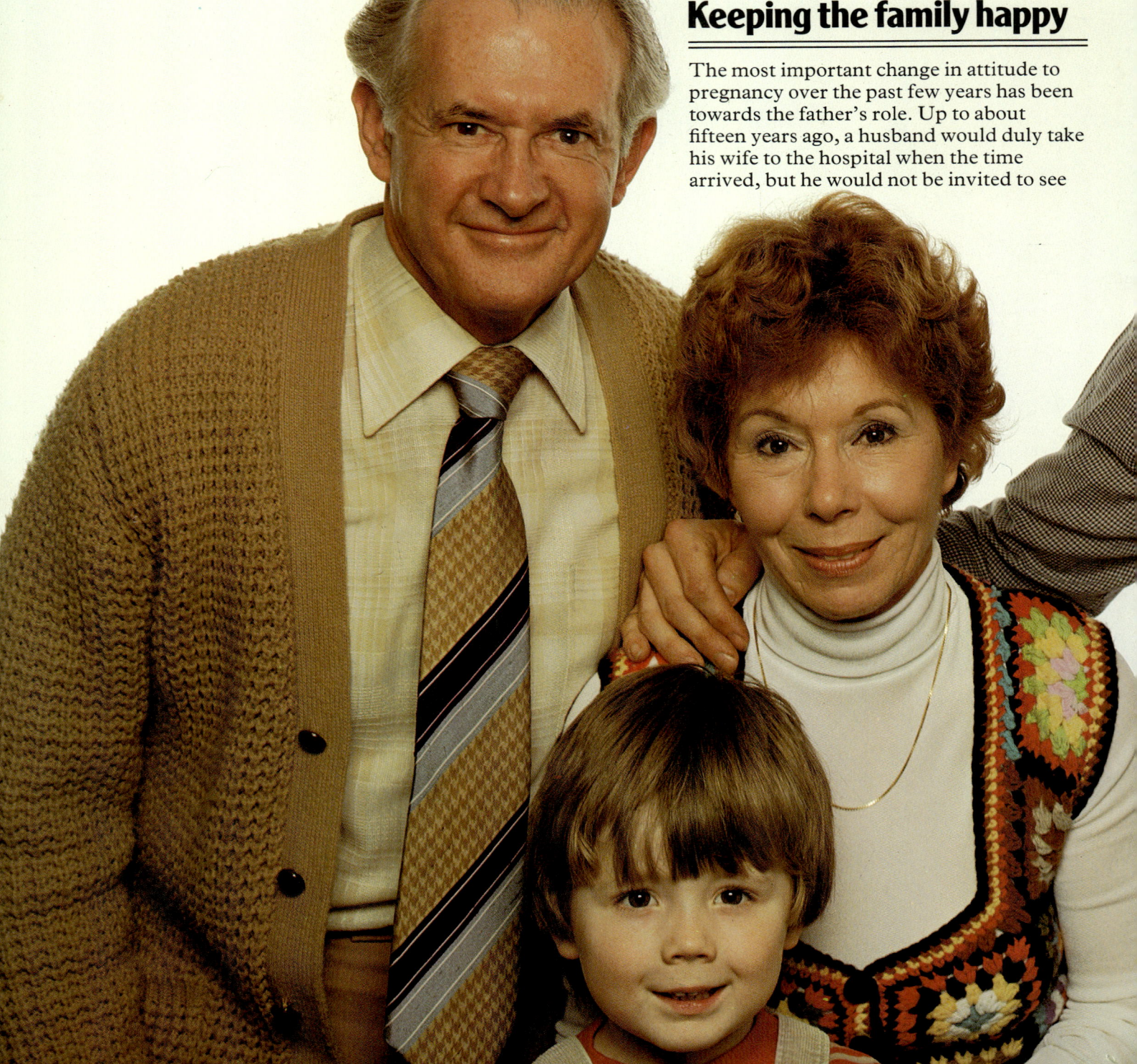

his child being born. Instead his first glimpse of the mother (fresh and clean in a new nightie) and baby (washed, swaddled and pink-cheeked) would probably be in the lying-in ward after the event.

Today most hospitals invite your partner to be with you at the birth. Many men indeed welcome the chance to be at the delivery and are fascinated by the mechanics of childbirth. However, it would be wrong to assume that because it is now fashionable to attend a birth every man automatically wants to join in. Some feel that they would not be able to cope with seeing their partner at such an emotional and perhaps overwrought time. Or they may find the physical aspect of childbirth distasteful. Alternatively, you yourself may feel that you can cope better in a more impersonal situation, without anyone very close to you being there. In general though, the more involved you allow your partner to become in your pregnancy the more likely you both are to want to share the experience of childbirth.

Men are now usually encouraged to

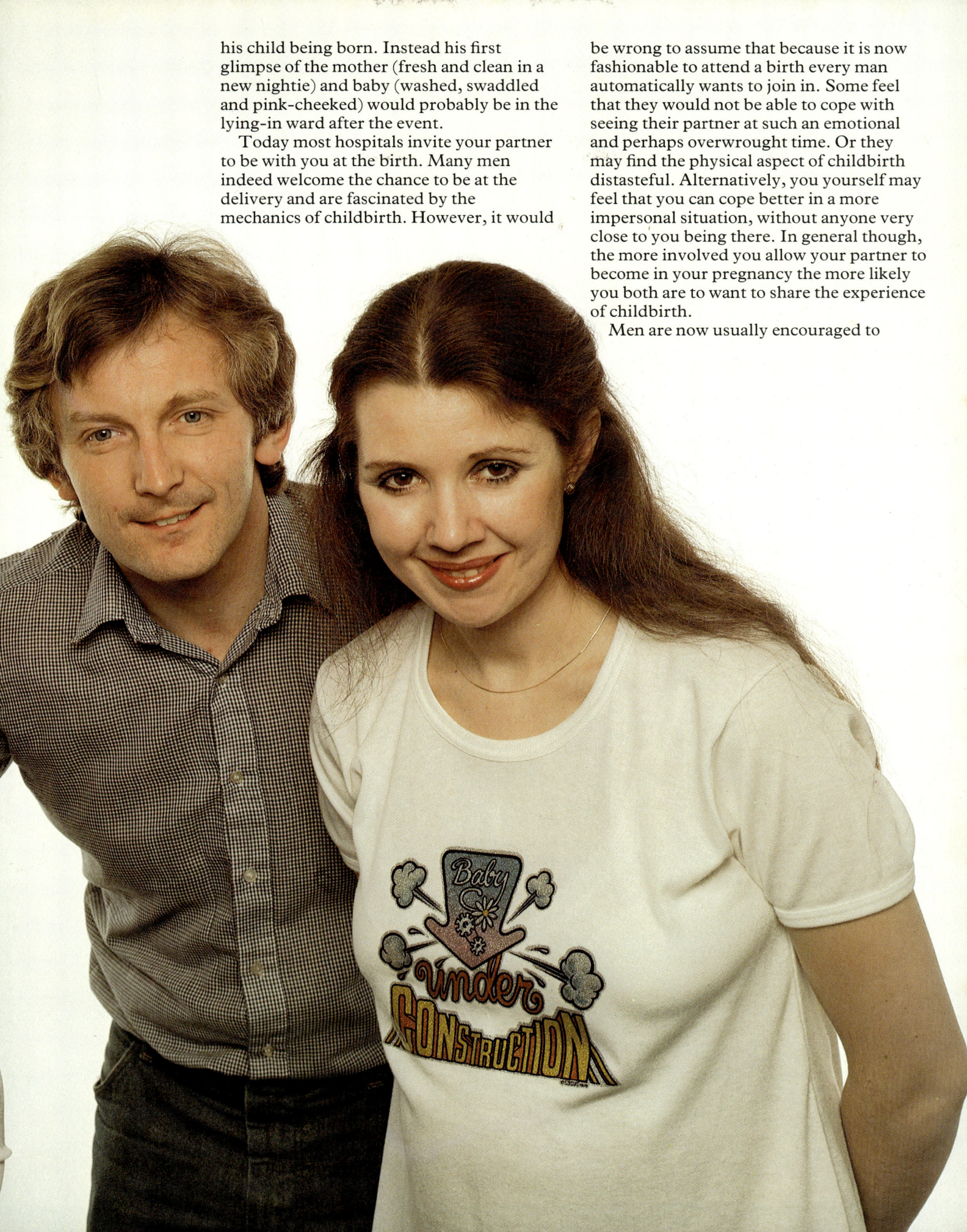

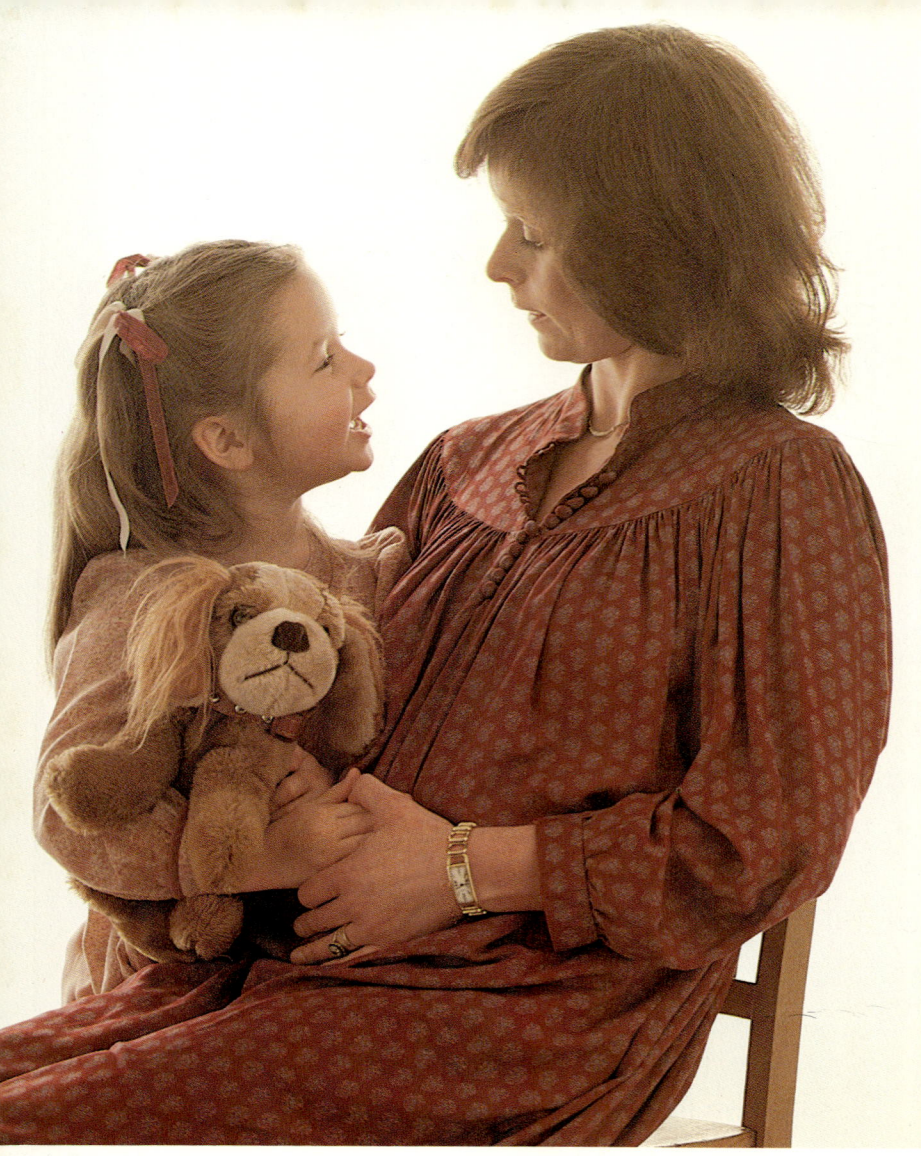

feels the baby moving he will get more used to the idea of having a new brother or sister, but he may well become bored with the waiting towards the end of your pregnancy.

You should prepare your child for the fact that the baby will do little but sleep and eat at first and that it will be some time before he is anything like the playmate and companion your child may expect. But stress that you will need lots of help and support when the baby is born so that he or she will feel involved in every stage of the baby's progress.

You may find yourself becoming irritated with well-meaning parents and in-laws who, with the best intentions, proffer unwanted advice and assistance. It's marvellous to have a mother or mother-in-law who can't wait for the birth of her grandchild and is standing by, ready to move in for a couple of weeks when you arrive home from hospital, especially if you are on your own. If you have come to this sort of arrangement you should each be quite sure what your roles will be. You will need someone to cook for you, perhaps to take your other children to school and collect them back again, do some shopping and generally pamper you a bit when you bring the baby home. What can lead to problems is a grandmother who wants only to look after the baby. That's your job unless you are looking for a nanny. Explain tactfully that it will be a real help if she can babysit at times but that in those early days after the birth it is you who needs looking after, just as much as the baby.

Older relatives may have different ideas about such domestic arrangements as where the baby should sleep, whether a man should change nappies, whether or not you should be thinking about leaving your child with a minder or in a crèche if you decide to go back to work. Try to deal with their arguments in a diplomatic but firm manner. You know how you want to organize your life and will have made your own plans. On the other hand, who wants to upset the family over minor domestic matters?

It is often assumed that a dog or cat is a certain threat to the new baby – perhaps the dog will be jealous and attack the baby or the cat sit on the baby and suffocate him. While these extreme possibilities are fairly unlikely there are steps you can take to avoid accidents. Discourage pets from going into the room you are preparing as the nursery before the baby is born. Buy a nylon catnet or large muslin square for the pram, and make sure that you never leave the baby alone with a cat or dog in the room.

Children are less likely to be jealous of a new baby if they have felt involved with the pregnancy.

attend antenatal classes and it can be a great help to have someone with you during labour to keep you occupied while you wait for something to happen, to remember your breathing exercises when you forget them in the heat of the moment and generally to provide moral support.

If you have an older child you may worry that he or she will be jealous of the new baby who is suddenly going to become the centre of attention. Introducing a new baby into the family has to be done tactfully and thoughtfully. There is bound to be some envy, but this can be minimized if you take the trouble to make your older child feel as loved and wanted as ever and keep him interested in what is going on.

Some mothers prefer not to mention their pregnancy until they are safely past the first three months or so when a miscarriage is more likely than at any other time. However, you should not delay telling your child too long if you don't want him or her to hear the news from anyone else.

As your child sees the growing bulge and

Have you remembered to...

CLAIM YOUR MATERNITY GRANT. Paid in a lump sum by Giro cheque, this can be claimed by all mothers on either the husband or wife's National Insurance. Claim on Form BM4 obtainable from a social security office, maternity or child welfare clinic at any time between fourteen weeks before the baby is expected and three months after he is born. You will also need to produce form MAT B1 – Certificate of Expected Confinement – which you can obtain from your doctor.

CLAIM YOUR MATERNITY ALLOWANCE. Mothers who have paid enough full insurance contributions while working either as an employee or for themselves are eligible for this. The allowance is payable for eighteen weeks starting eleven weeks before the baby is due, but cannot be drawn for any weeks during this period when you are doing paid work. Claim on form BM4 between fourteen and eleven weeks before the baby is expected. If you claim after the eleventh week the allowance cannot be backdated.

CLAIM MATERNITY PAY. Find out if you have worked for your employer long enough to be eligible for maternity pay. If so, you are required to work up to the eleventh week before your baby is due, and must notify your employer at least three weeks before you leave that you are doing so because you are pregnant. If you are entitled to maternity leave and want to take this, you must at the same time inform your employer of your intention to return to work and give the expected date of your confinement.

CLAIM ADDITIONAL MATERNITY BENEFITS. Find out from any social security office if you can claim additional maternity benefits – for example, if you have twins or a multiple birth. You may also be eligible for an increased allowance if you are a one-parent family or your husband is unable to support himself through physical disability.

MAKE USE OF FREE SERVICES. Make sure you have any necessary dental treatment – it is free for expectant mothers and women who have a child up to a year old. The same goes for prescription charges. You may also be entitled to free glasses and dentures on the National Health Service and, in a few areas, chiropody. Again, enquire at your local social security office.

FIND OUT ABOUT NUTRITIONAL BENEFITS. Under certain circumstances you may be able to claim free milk and vitamins – ask at your social security office, child welfare or maternity clinic.

Organizing the household

Good planning is essential when you have a family and if you start getting into a routine when you are pregnant, say, doing big shopping trips monthly and having specific times for housework, you should find that this will help a great deal when the baby ties you down to a schedule.

As housework and shopping become more difficult towards the end of pregnancy, try to organize yourself so that you have fewer trips to make to the shops and more time to relax. Clear out a cupboard for stores of tinned foods and such essentials as soap, toothpaste, toilet paper, and so on, and do one big shop at a supermarket or cash-and-carry to stock up for several weeks. If you have one, a freezer is a tremendous bonus – during the last month of pregnancy you can fill it with sufficient meat, fish, vegetables and so on to see you through until some time after the birth. If you can afford it, and are lucky enough to find one, a lady who will come in for two or three hours a week to give the house a real clean out is invaluable, especially if later she can be relied on to keep an eye on the baby while you do some shopping. If you do the housework yourself, try to keep everything generally as free from mess and clutter as possible and set aside a couple of mornings a week to dust, vacuum, change bed linen and wash floors. As long as you keep the house manageably tidy there is no need for exhaustive dusting and cleaning every day.

Electrical gadgets may seem expensive and noisy but many do have their advantages. A blender or liquidizer, for instance, will save time and elbow grease in making soups, sauces and desserts. And, when your baby is old enough for solid foods, you can save money by puréeing small portions of family meals rather than buying expensive baby foods. If you are thinking of buying a washing machine to cope with all the nappies and baby clothes, it's as well to take delivery two or three months before your baby is expected.

When the Big Day Arrives

The last month of pregnancy is invariably an interminable period of waiting for something to happen, filled with excitement, apprehension, last minute doubts and plain boredom. The date of delivery your doctor has given you is an estimate based on the length of the average pregnancy, so there is an eighty-five per cent chance that you could have your baby in the two weeks preceding the expected date, and unfortunately there is also an eighty-five per cent chance that you could be hanging on for an extra fortnight, so don't depend on the baby arriving on the day. Friends phoning you to ask 'are you still here?' can seem the last straw, and it is a good idea to make social plans past the date you have been given so that you aren't left with too much time on your hands if you are late. After all, you have an excellent reason to cancel if need be.

Recognizing the onset of labour

Some women worry that they may not recognize the signs of their labour starting or fear that they might have a false alarm – something that does quite often happen. The uterus in fact contracts every fifteen to twenty minutes throughout pregnancy, although this is not felt as anything other than a tightening of the abdomen until towards the end of term. During the last six weeks, the contractions may be felt as a vaguely uncomfortable sensation, not unlike that of a mild period pain. These are often called 'practice contractions' and are sometimes misinterpreted as the onset of labour. There are however three classic and very recognizable symptoms of the beginning of labour which, once you know what to expect, cannot be mistaken.

The rupture of the membranes (breaking of the waters), is painless and feels like a popping sensation, apparently in the anus. If the baby's head hasn't yet engaged (see page 13) you may lose a larger quantity of

fluid from the vagina than if it has. But in either event it will probably be quite a noticeable amount. Although you will be unlikely to start labour contractions for anything up to twelve hours, you should phone the hospital immediately for instructions as to when to come in.

The second classic sign is to have a 'show' – that is a small amount of pinkish blood mixed with mucus. This is quite normal and associated with the dislodgement of the 'plug' (a solid lump of clear, sticky mucus) from the cervix, which occurs before the onset of labour or in its first stages.

Finally, you may experience powerful, regular contractions of the uterus. These are more frequent than practice contractions and last longer – a minute or two at a time. They could be felt as a low, nagging backache together with a tightening of the abdomen or with strong cramps in the abdomen itself, sometimes described as similar to severe period pains, or sharp discomfort accompanying diarrhoea.

Preparations you should have made

For the baby
The baby's requirements should have been thought out by the last month and his sleeping quarters organized. You will probably receive many items as gifts and you can fill in gaps after your stay in hospital, but the following is a check list of what you will need right from the start:

Three stretch baby suits (these can be used for day and night, or buy nighties if you prefer); three vests, three cardigans; a shawl; booties, mittens and helmets if your baby is born in winter; bibs; two or three pairs of waterproof pants; two dozen terry towelling nappies plus muslin squares or disposable nappy liners; pins; nappy rash cream; bottles and sterilizing equipment; lots of cotton wool and tissues.

The baby's room should be aired thoroughly and then kept warm – a

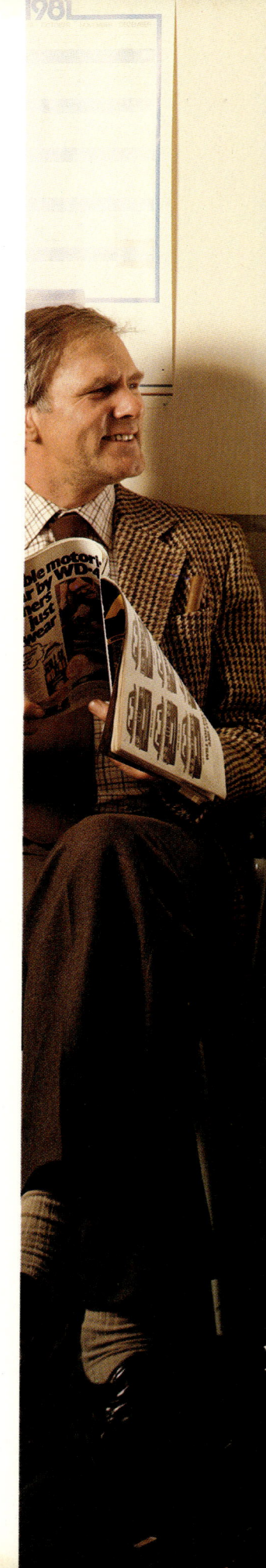

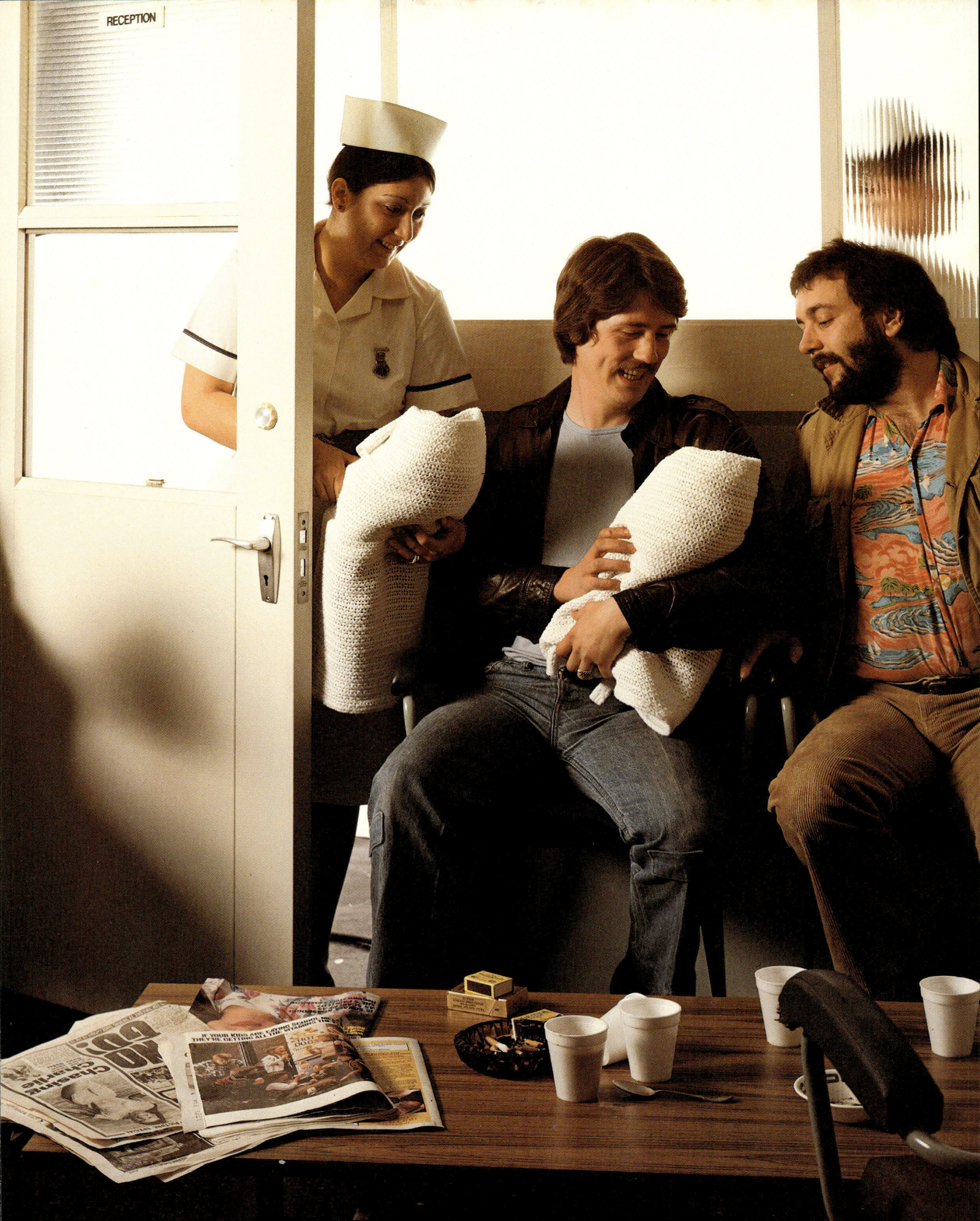

temperature of 60° to 65°F (15° to 18°C). He can sleep in a carry-cot or crib at first or go straight into a standard-sized cot (a carry-cot of course can double as a cot and a pram). Always make sure that any equipment has the British Standard 'Kitemark' for safety. You will need flanelette sheets, blankets and a waterproof undersheet for the baby's bed, though not a pillow, also a baby bath, two bath towels, baby soap, and a soft hairbrush. Other useful equipment is a baby chair and/or high chair, and a carry-cot pram.

For yourself

It is essential to have a suitcase packed and ready with everything you need for the delivery and your stay in hospital from the thirty-sixth week of pregnancy onwards. If you do go into labour early and have to leave home in a rush, you want to be sure that you haven't forgotten anything.

Leave out a set of clean clothes that can be brought to the hospital for your return and make sure that whoever is picking you up knows where they are. You should be able to get into some of your old clothes straight away but don't be tempted to pack anything that is tight or waisted. Try and get into your jeans and you'll be disappointed – it takes a few weeks of exercise to get your figure back into shape. Also you will feel tender, especially if you have had stitches, and struggling into an unwilling pair of trousers will only make things worse.

With everything at home organized all you have to do is wait. If your partner is going to be with you at the birth or take you to hospital, you must know where to contact him at all times. If you have to rely on yourself to get to the hospital and don't need an ambulance (these should only be called in an emergency) never attempt to drive, or take public transport, but keep the number of a reliable cab firm handy at all times. Don't forget your hospital admission card and antenatal notes if you have been given them.

Do try to keep busy during those last few weeks. You may well feel like just sitting around the house waiting for something to happen, but thinking about the delivery unfortunately won't bring it on any faster. Relax – and let the start of your labour be a pleasant surprise rather than a tensely anticipated event.

Have your suitcase packed in good time so that you are all ready to go if the baby arrives early.

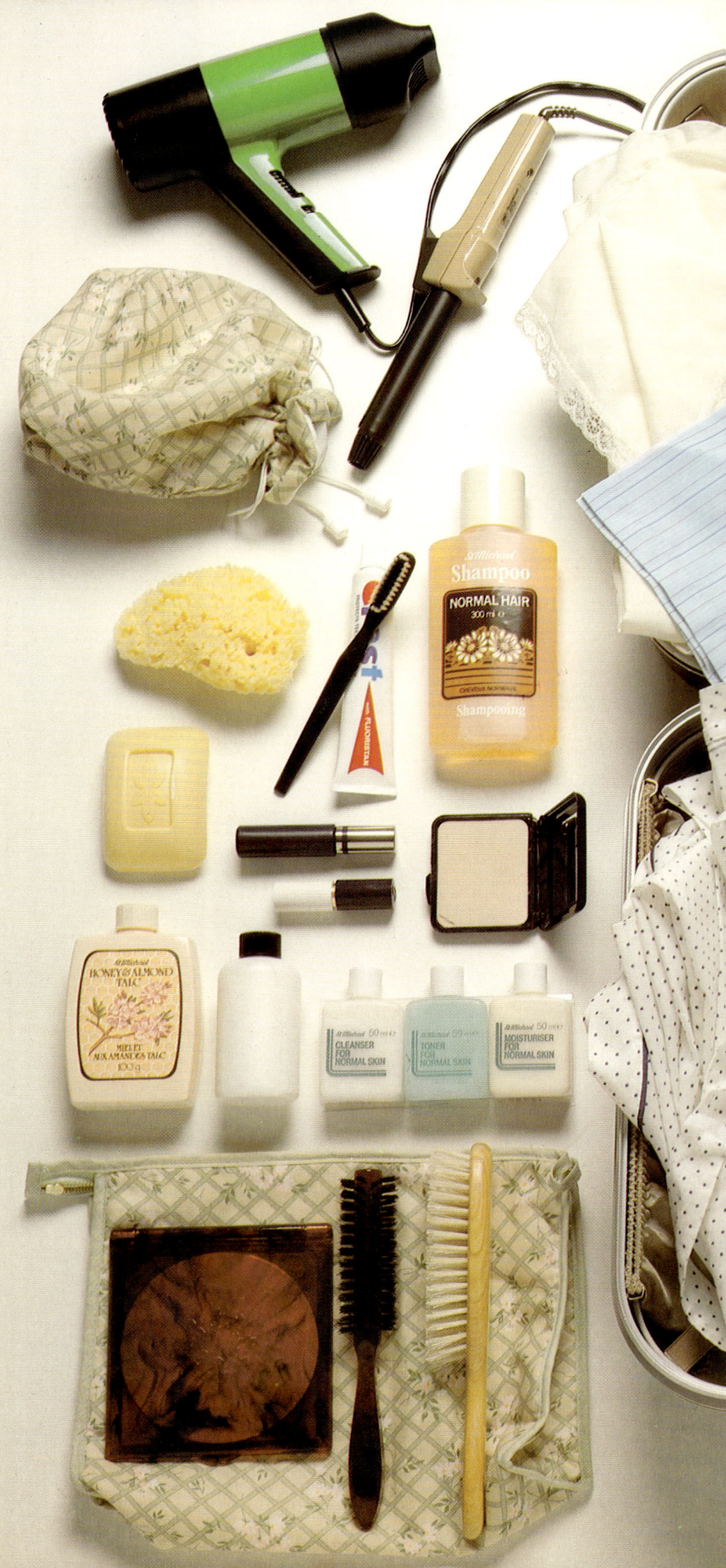

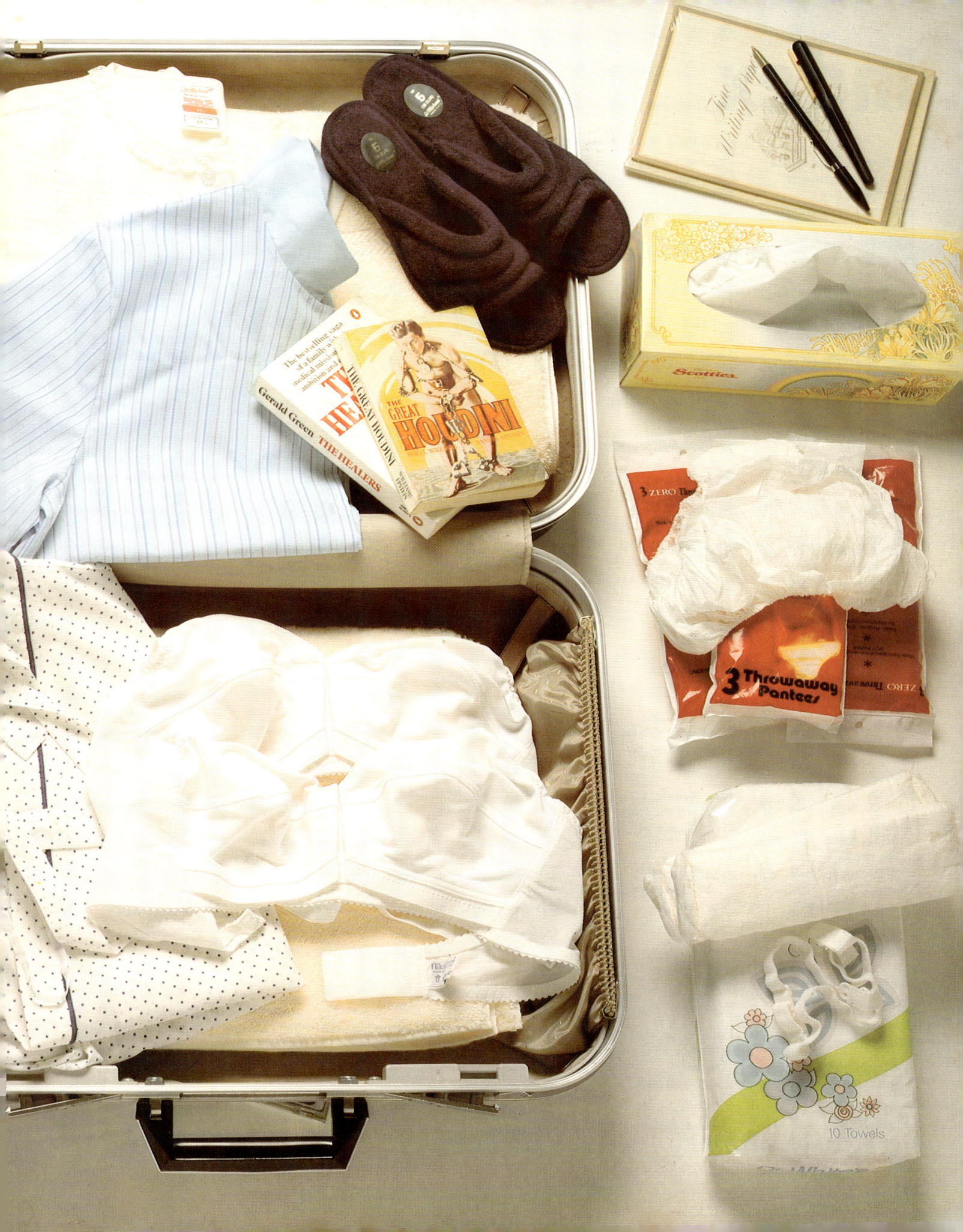